succeeding

as a

nurse

the experts share
their secrets

foreword by Beverly Malone

HEALTH PRESS

Succeeding as a Nurse
First published April 2005

© 2005 in this edition Health Press Limited
Health Press Limited, Elizabeth House, Queen Street, Abingdon,
Oxford OX14 3LN, UK
Tel: +44 (0)1235 523233
Fax: +44 (0)1235 523238

A CIP catalogue record for this title is available from the British Library.

ISBN 1-903734-69-X

Health Press thanks all those involved in the production of this book – notably the
contributors, for their ongoing commitment; Professor Dame June Clark, for her work
in the early stages; the nurse reviewers, for their helpful advice and comments; Tricia Reid,
for her work on the 'key skills' chapters; and Dr Laura Price, for her editorial direction,
project management and 'making it happen'.

Typesetting and page layout by Zed, Oxford, UK.
Printed by Linney*print*, Mansfield, UK.

Printed with vegetable-oil-based inks on fully biodegradable and
recyclable paper manufactured from sustainable forests.

Contents

Career destinations

Foreword

I am delighted to support this new book for nurses. By reading it, you are giving yourself permission to succeed as a nurse, and that's an important step. There has never been a more exciting time to be in nursing, or a greater need for quality care.

Today, many people from increasingly diverse backgrounds are coming into nursing from other careers, often starting out as healthcare assistants. Diploma- and degree-level study is the norm and two in ten nurses have a degree. Many nurses practise beyond NHS hospitals – in the independent sector, community care, business and government. There are many challenging, rewarding career destinations on offer.

The new NHS pay and careers system is set to reward nurses for the demanding and complex work we do. The Knowledge and Skills Framework will help to enhance lifelong learning as well as providing gateways for career progression.

Choosing to succeed will have a positive impact on the patients and communities you serve. Solid evidence is mounting about the positive impact of nursing on patients' experience and perception of healthcare as well as reductions in patient mortality, medication errors and patient falls.

Getting a quality deal for patients and nurses motivates me on my own nursing journey, spanning practice, education, research, management, professional activism and leadership. Nurses are, and always will be, vital to shaping and delivering quality, accessible and person-centred care. Read on to learn about the skills you need as you prepare to succeed as a nurse.

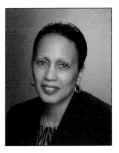

Beverly Malone,
General Secretary,
Royal College of Nursing

Introduction

Succeeding as a Nurse is the third book in the 'Succeeding as...' series. In these books, our aim is to couple helpful information with advice and tips from people who really know what they're talking about. The ones doing the jobs. Caring for patients, working with colleagues, managing teams.

In this book, the first chapters deal with the 'key skills' you need as a modern nurse. For example: how to handle difficult situations; how to make an effective presentation; how to work well in a team.

And then we're delighted that in the second part of the book, which we've called 'Career destinations', we've been able to include chapters from nurses in a wide cross-section of roles. Of course, we haven't been able to cover every role – nothing like it – but we hope the selection that we have included will highlight the variety of career pathways that are open to you as a nurse. And if you already know where you're going, or indeed you're well on the way, we hope that you still enjoy hearing about the ups and downs that go with the different name badges.

The book ends with a contribution from journalist Tricia Reid. Unlike our other contributors, Tricia doesn't have a nursing background, but she did spend 4 years as Editor of the *Nursing Times*, so she knows what she's talking about.

We hope you enjoy our book and that it helps you achieve success, however you want to define it.

The Health Press team

We'd be glad to hear what you thought of this book, and we particularly welcome suggestions for improvement. Please contact us at post@healthpress.co.uk

key skills

"always bear in mind that your own resolution
to succeed is more important than any one thing"
Abraham Lincoln
16th president of the USA (1809–1865)

getting the most out of training

Education and training for nurses does not stop with the end of the initial training period. 'Professional development', 'continuing education' and 'lifelong learning' are hot phrases that you are going to hear throughout your career (and they crop up quite a lot in this book, too). If you want to progress, you will have to do a range of ongoing training relevant to your chosen specialty.

The world of nursing is in a constant state of flux and change. Government targets and advances in medicine and medical procedures mean there is a constant need to update your practice. There are also many more opportunities for nurses to take on senior roles within the wider healthcare team.

When you started out you may have had an image of a nurse working in a hospital. But you could find yourself working in a GP surgery, a specialist clinic, a nursing or residential home, occupational health services, a voluntary organization that runs a hospice, residential care or the pharmaceutical industry. And of course nurses also work in the armed services, prisons, schools and the leisure industry.

A new era

The range of responsibilities that nurses have has also changed dramatically over the years, sometimes controversially. Nurses can now prescribe a range of drugs and dressings. Some nurses now carry out a range of procedures previously only carried out by doctors. Nurses could soon be trained to perform surgery to help reduce hospital waiting lists. Under the government's plans, a wide range of operations, including hernia repair,

there are **many opportunities** to take on **senior roles** vasectomies and arthroscopies will be performed by surgical care practitioners – some of whom will be qualified nurses – after 2 years of training. Plans are afoot to appoint up to 5000 over the next decade.

What is expected of you

As a nurse it is your responsibility to update your knowledge and practice. The speed of change in the delivery of healthcare means that the Department of Health has been at pains to develop a culture of lifelong learning among its staff. As a nurse you are often the first point of contact for patients, and updating your practice is a vital and legal responsibility laid down by your regulatory body, the Nursing and Midwifery Council (NMC). It is the NMC's duty to protect the public by setting professional standards and providing guidance to nurses and midwives as to how to meet them.

it is your responsibility to update your practice

Postregistration education and practice (PREP) is a set of standards laid down by the NMC which allows you to demonstrate that you are keeping up to date and building on your knowledge and skills. They are legal requirements. You have to re-register to practise every 3 years by submitting a signed notification of practice form which asks you to declare that you have met the standards. You cannot re-register unless you have met the standards and can prove it. There are two standards which must be met: the PREP (practice) standard and the PREP (continuing professional development [CPD]) standard.

The PREP (practice) standard

The PREP (practice) standard requires you to have worked as a nurse for a minimum of 100 days in the previous 5 years. If you have not done this, you will have to successfully complete a return-to-practice course. You can meet the standard whether you are in full-time work or work part-time. You can even fulfil it if you have not worked for a while – perhaps you've been caring for children or a close relative. You can also fulfil it if you have been working as a volunteer, as long as you can provide evidence that the experience you have gained is relevant to the work you are doing or hope to do.

The PREP (CPD) standard

The PREP (CPD) standard requires you to record in a personal professional portfolio how you have kept up to date over the 3 years prior to renewing your registration. You

you can decide how you want to meet the standard

must complete the equivalent of 5 days or 35 hours of learning activity. The NMC has been under pressure from various fronts to state what are approved PREP learning activities. So far it has resisted the temptation to be prescriptive. This means you can decide how you want to meet the standard and do it in a way that suits your own learning style. There is no approved format for the portfolio either, and you don't have to collect academic points or certificates of attendance at conferences and courses. And there is no special folder you should keep your work in, although there are some on the market. A normal loose-leaf file will do.

There is a wide range of activities that will help you meet the standards.

- You could read something related to your practice in an academic journal and write a short reflection on what you learned from it and how you will apply it in your practice.
- You could write something for a professional journal (see page 32).
- You could attend a course run by your trust or an outside organization.
- You could attend a conference relevant to your clinical work.
- You could write a piece of reflective work on your experience of caring for a specific patient.
- You could act as a preceptor or mentor.

The important thing is that you record what you have done so that you can prove it if the NMC asks you to do so. So it is vital to start keeping a professional portfolio now, if you have not already done so.

The NMC offers guidance on the type of information you should supply in your professional portfolio (Table 1). But there are no hard and fast rules. The PREP handbook, published by the NMC, offers a template to help you ensure you include the right information.

Clinical supervision

Clinical supervision is another phrase you will hear a lot throughout your career and it is a big part of your lifelong learning and ongoing training and development. Basically, it is a bit like mentorship – it brings practitioners and supervisors together to reflect on practice, discuss problems and come up with solutions.

Clinical supervision is developed at local level and should not be confused with the appraisal process. Your supervisor does not have to be your line manager. It should be training and learning experience for the supervisee and it is an integral part of lifelong learning. If you work somewhere where it is not offered as a formal support mechanism you should be asking why.

The NMC has defined a set of principles that should shape clinical supervision in any healthcare environment.

- It should support your practice, enabling you to maintain and improve standards of care.
- It should be a practice-focused professional relationship, involving a practitioner.
- It should allow you to reflect on practice guided by a skilled supervisor.

- Ground rules should be agreed so that you and your supervisor approach clinical supervision openly and confidently and you are both aware of what is involved.

The NMC advises that principles and relevance of clinical supervision should be included in preregistration and postregistration education programmes. Evaluation of clinical supervision is needed to assess how it influences care and practice standards. Evaluation systems should be determined locally.

Ongoing training

One relatively recent development in the NHS has been the launch of the NHS University (NHSU) in October 2003. The NHSU was born out of a 4-month consultation that showed training and development opportunities across the NHS to be patchy. Awareness of what is available is often low, and accessing courses can be difficult.

Unfortunately, the NHSU has been a short-lived innovation. Its dissolution at the end of July 2005 leaves a gap that is being filled by the NHS Institute for Learning Skills and Innovation. These changes are part of the Secretary of State's bureaucracy-cutting exercise to free money for frontline services.

The good news is that the government is committed to staff training – and training is actually happening! The 2004 NHS staff survey found that 93% of staff received some kind of training, up from 89% in the 2003 survey. So if you're not getting it, ask why.

A framework for lifelong learning was published by the NHS in 2001. *Working Together, Learning Together* aims to improve patient care and expand NHS career opportunities. It sets out targets for financial and cultural investment in a lifelong learning culture, and sets an agenda for stakeholders. The framework is aimed at education providers and employers, so the onus is on them to provide you with the kind of training you need.

Nursing is full of many specialties, although there are generic courses you can access, such as using information technology and handling violent patients. The best way to access the training that is right for you is through discussion at your appraisal. Your trust will usually respond to demand – and to instructions from government. But it's a good idea to come up with a few suggestions for what you want.

There are a number of training providers – independent providers and universities. You could join one of the RCN specialist forums, which allows you to network with others doing your kind of work. There is also the RCN Institute, which offers flexible distance-learning programmes if you want to get an academic qualification.

You might like to take a look at the Unison Open College, which can be accessed through their website. They offer a range of courses, provided by themselves and by outside organizations.

Knowledge and Skills Framework

At the heart of how you tackle the issue of your own ongoing training is the NHS Knowledge and Skills Framework (KSF). The KSF is a tool providing a means of recognizing the broad skills and knowledge that a person needs to apply to be effective in a particular NHS post. The KSF will be applicable across the range of NHS posts covered by Agenda for Change, ensuring better links between education, development, career and pay progression.

The aim of KSF is that staff will:

- have clear and consistent development objectives
- be helped to develop in such a way that they can apply the knowledge and skills appropriate to their job
- be helped to identify and develop knowledge and skills that will support their career progression and encourage lifelong learning.

Staff should receive annual development reviews provided by their line manager and they will be able to agree personal development plans. The KSF describes health, safety and security as a key aspect of all jobs to which Agenda for Change applies. It makes it clear that it is vital that everyone takes responsibility for promoting the health, safety and security of patients and clients, the public, colleagues and themselves.

one of the ways in which staff progress is by being more proactive

The KSF describes how, as staff move forward in their careers, their responsibilities for activities connected with health, safety and security also progress and the different levels of competence required. One of the ways in which staff progress is by being more proactive and more focused on good practice and going from following set procedures to identifying the need for improvement.

Making this a key aspect of all jobs covered by the NHS KSF will help to raise staff's awareness of their immediate and continuing responsibility for good practice – in general hygiene, for example, which is a big issue for nurses given the whole MRSA debacle. Chris Beasley, the Chief Nursing Officer in England, has announced that over one million NHS staff are to receive training to help in the fight against MRSA.

An all-graduate profession

There has been heated debate over the past decade as to whether nursing should be an all-graduate profession. If you are going to study for 3 or 4 years, as most undergraduates do, then why should you not get the hat and gown treatment at the end of it?

By now you will know only too well that you can go the degree or diploma route to qualify as a nurse. If you have a diploma and you want a degree, then you can easily get one by picking up some modules at university. This allows you to be flexible on the amount of time you want to spend studying, and will let you spread the load over a timeframe to suit you.

Further reading

Information about Unison's Learning and Organising Services are available from www.unison.org.uk/laos

Department of Health. *Working Together, Learning Together: A Framework for Lifelong Learning for the NHS.* London: TSO, 2001 (available from www.dh.gov.uk).

Nursing and Midwifery Council. *Supporting Nurses and Midwives Through Lifelong Learning.* London: Nursing and Midwifery Council, 2002 (available from www.nmc-uk.org).

Nursing and Midwifery Council. *The PREP Handbook.* London, Nursing and Midwifery Council, 2004 (available from www.nmc-uk.org).

working effectively

Working as part of a team

In the modern NHS, nurses are no longer a homogeneous group who carry out a set of defined tasks. They are individual team players who carry a range of responsibilities and have numerous skills they can bring to the wider healthcare team. For example, pain management nurses work alongside consultant oncologists and radiotherapists to provide the range of care a cancer patient needs. And in many cases, clinical nurse specialists, nurse consultants and nurse practitioners lead healthcare teams. Enlightened medical colleagues accept this. The time of seeing nurses at the beck and call of doctors is well and truly over.

Characteristics of good teams

Effective clinical teams should, of course, put patients first, and possess a number of key characteristics (Table 2). In particular, successful teams should be able to demonstrate:

- purpose and value, including evidence of leadership, well-defined values, standards, functions and responsibilities and strategic direction
- performance, including evidence of competent management, good systems, good performance records, effective internal performance monitoring, feedback and regular appraisal; in addition, all team members should accept responsibility for their own and each other's performance
- consistency, including evidence of thoroughness and a systematic approach to patient care
- effectiveness and efficiency, including evidence of thorough medical and clinical audit that the clinical team is continually assessing its care and outcomes
- a chain of responsibility, including evidence that the responsibilities of each of the team members are well defined and understood

- openness, such as a willingness for transparency to others, evidence of comparative external review, and performance measures that can be easily understood by those outside the team
- overall acceptability, including evidence that the overall performance and results achieved by the team inspire the trust and confidence of patients, employers and professional colleagues.

Delegation skills

How you carry out your role as part of the healthcare team is all down to your clinical credibility and your communication skills. You need to know what to do and how to do it – and you need to be able to tell others. You also need to be able to delegate appropriately. Delegation is not only the right of the person at the top of the pecking order. As a nurse you are in a position to delegate tasks you are not skilled to do or are just too busy for. All good teams will have access to healthcare assistants. These people are trained and skilled to carry out basic nursing tasks, so freeing up qualified staff to carry out more complex tasks and ensuring that the patients get an all-round good care experience.

Don't confuse delegation with bossing someone about. Healthcare assistants are what their role says they are, but they are no more your dogsbody than you are the doctor's. The role of the healthcare assistant is a sensitive one. Many have several years' experience and may know more than you if you are a fairly new nurse. There has been a significant amount of campaigning on their behalf to have their skills recognized and their role in the team acknowledged.

To delegate effectively, you will need to have a good relationship with your team members – not one based on superiority. Remember that those you stab in the back on your way up the ladder may get their revenge when you are on the way down!

A good approach

Take a close look at the others in the team and the way in which they interact. Make sure you are completely sure of everyone's role. There should be a feeling of mutual confidence among all the team players. Disagreements within healthcare teams usually come down to assumptions about what someone should be doing, or ignorance of what their role is. But if someone is not pulling their weight, you are unlikely to be the only team member who has noticed.

However, this is not an excuse to gang up on someone. If you feel that someone interacts badly, even if it is someone more senior than you, you should find a way to address the issue. Ask a senior member of the team to clarify everyone's role for you. If the matter which concerns you is a skills issue which could affect patient care then this is more serious and you must report it to the team leader or, if the issue is associated with this person, to the director of nursing or the human resources manager. You've got to be brave to do it. But think how you would feel if a patient was harmed while you stood idly by.

Because of the nature of the work you do, where things have to happen quickly and effectively, it is not always possible to save someone's feelings. But you don't have to be rude. Good team players have tact. If there is a good rapport, minor mistakes can be highlighted through humour. Say what you think tactfully, having thought the matter through. Openness and honesty are crucial for effective team working.

Managing your time

It's a sad fact that nurses never seem to have enough time to do anything to their complete satisfaction. There may be more nurses working in the

NHS than ever before, but few at the coal face would say they've noticed. Nurses particularly complain that they never have enough time to talk to patients. As nurses are often the health professionals who are the first point of contact for patients, this is not a good situation.

It is estimated that 80% of a person's productivity is a result of 20% of his or her time. If this is true, most of our time is wasted. Some people are perfectionists and will achieve less because of their quest for perfection in everything they do. On balance, efficiency is better than perfection for most purposes, and becomes all the more important when your workload increases.

Your time is not your own. You can plan your time all you like, but it is dictated by the often urgent and unexpected health needs of the patients, who do not deteriorate or get better to fit with your workload. You can manage your time better if you set priorities, paying particular attention to tasks that only you can perform, and stick to them. One of the most important time management skills to acquire is successful delegation. Does the task really need a nurse to do it? If a healthcare assistant is available and could do a task as well, if not better, than you, then delegate if it is appropriate to do so. But be realistic. Everyone is busy, and you should accept that you cannot plan in any degree of detail.

efficiency is better than perfection for most purposes

Try to avoid starting something that you are not going to finish. Whenever possible, complete one task before moving on to the next. It's also unwise to postpone an unpleasant or boring task. Best to get it out of the way – it will never improve with time.

Paperwork

Don't let paperwork build up. The bane of every nurse's life is patient records and what a mess they usually are. Paperwork is only of value if it contains useful information. Fill in patient records as you complete tasks. Don't put it off until later, when you will have forgotten or got the patient mixed up with someone else. Patient records are crucial to good patient care.

By the time you read this, it is possible that you will have access to electronic patient records. The NHS is going through something of an IT revolution and the government has set itself a target of 2007 for health professionals to be able to access patient records from a central database.

You need to be an expert and meticulous record-keeper. Patient records are the most precious resource available to you if you are to carry out your job properly and appropriately. They are also the one thing that can act against you if you fail to fill them out properly. You are legally required to time, date and sign entries you make on a patient's records, indeed any paperwork you produce as part of your job, be it a note to the consultant or patient advice.

Most members of the team will have access to and will write in a patient's notes. So it's common sense to make sure someone can read and understand whatever you write. Over the years there has been a clampdown on sloppy note-taking. Doctors for years have had a reputation for appalling handwriting! Be careful and meticulous. And resist the temptation to write derogatory comments about a patient. Some people might find it funny to write SOS (silly old sod) or COT (cantankerous old twit) in someone's notes. But it will not be tolerated, is highly unprofessional and could land you in trouble. You also run the risk of losing your credibility with other colleagues, not to mention your job.

there has been a clampdown on sloppy note-taking

The phone

Nurses have to talk to colleagues all the time, but making telephone calls is another potentially time-wasting activity when you have only a one in four chance of reaching the person you want to speak to. Make the most of email where you can. Nurses working in the community are increasingly using email to plan and communicate their caseloads to other colleagues and, as they're all equipped with mobile phones, they also use text. A useful resource when you are with your patients and don't want to be distracted.

You may not have access to email on the ward, but forward-thinking trusts encourage the use of it, and provide email addresses to their staff. Email is part of our lives now – even if you only use it to tell sister you're sick it's worth embracing it. It's much more direct than the phone sometimes, and people also tend to read it and respond immediately. It also, of course, provides a timed and dated record of what has been communicated.

The people who manage their time best are those who can say 'no'. Be assertive but not aggressive. And don't waste time trying to get your head around something you don't understand. Be prepared to ask for clarification and advice or information from others when you need it.

Finally, while this is all about making time in your day to talk to patients, you also need to make time to think about the bigger picture and spend time developing your own personal career strategy. Decide what your goals are and set yourself a realistic timeframe within which to achieve them. Where do you want to be, and when? Carefully consider the potential pitfalls and identify what your key focus areas should be. Regularly take the time to think about your career strategy and constantly modify it as individual goals are achieved.

Asserting yourself

If you want to get on in nursing, you must get yourself noticed. You can do this in a variety of ways. To get noticed you must assert yourself, but don't confuse assertion with aggression. No one likes the pushy, bossy one.

Make sure you get to know as much as possible about how your organization is run. Who does what? Who has power and influence? Which is the most effective department and why? This all keys in to where you want to be in the organization and in your career. You are planning your route.

If you have a good idea, or if something particularly positive has happened in your area of work, tell people. Email the communications director – and copy it to the chief executive. No one ever got sacked for telling good news.

Get some leadership skills

All nurses need leadership skills (see Table 3). You have to lead yourself (quite often you are working alone) and you have to offer leadership to staff who are junior to you. You may not see yourself as a leader, but people who want to learn from you do.

The Department of Health seriously encourages the development of leadership skills at all levels of the NHS, so much so that it has developed the Leadership Centre to devise programmes that allow nurses and other

Table 3

Leadership skills: attributes of good practice

- Take the initiative to ensure the team is involved
- If necessary, take command of the situation and advocate your own position
- Consider other people's suggestions
- Motivate the team through appreciation and provide coaching when necessary
- Adopt standard protocols and ensure the team complies
- Intervene if the team's performance deviates from standards
- Justify deviations from standard procedures when necessary following consultation with the team
- Demonstrate the intention to achieve the highest possible standard under the prevailing conditions
- Encourage your team to participate in planning and completing tasks
- Ensure that the plan is clearly stated, together with the goals and boundaries for completing it
- Change the plan if necessary after consulting with the team
- Allocate tasks to team members, and check and correct as appropriate
- Prioritize secondary, operational tasks to retain sufficient resources to meet the primary objectives
- Allow sufficient time to complete tasks
- In an emergency, off-load – delegate the tasks that can be safely accomplished by junior team members (even if they will perform these tasks less well than more senior colleagues), in order to free more experienced team members to consider wider issues and to supervise the effort of the whole team
- Appreciate and allow for a down turn in performance because of stress or fatigue

healthcare professionals to develop a career path. You don't need to be top of the tree to be a good leader. But you do need to be a confident and efficient practitioner.

The Royal College of Nursing (RCN) also has its own government-funded clinical leadership programme linked to the Leadership Centre. It aims to develop individuals and teams, develop patient focus, and enhance networking and political awareness. Over 2000 people have already completed the programme. It is aimed at nurses and other healthcare professionals who have a responsibility to lead clinical care. Just think – one day it may be you.

Working independently

Nurses are always part of a wider team, but many spend a lot of time working on their own, especially if they are working in the community. Managing your own caseload and workload can be very liberating, but it can be nerve wracking too. You will have to make many decisions without the guidance of a colleague, often going on your gut instinct.

You must make sure you work within the realms of your capabilities. If you are faced with a problem with a patient and you are unsure what to do, you should hang fire until you can speak to a more senior or experienced colleague. For example, if you are visiting an elderly patient to treat a leg ulcer, and they insist that they do not want the wound dressed, what would you do? Your instinct may be to persuade the elderly lady to let you do what you know to be good for her. But then you may end up with a complaint on your hands from a disgruntled daughter who says you bullied her mother. Make sure you think things through.

You should away make sure you practise to the best of your abilities to protect yourself and your patients. Time pressures mean that it is all too easy to cut corners. Nurses are constantly working under time constraints. It comes with the territory. But someone's health could be put at risk on the basis of a decision you make when under pressure. Supposing you have four home visits to do. Mr Bloggs was okay yesterday, so perhaps you can give him a miss today. Really, you should make sure you are where you are supposed to be, even if you are running late. But in this instance, you may miss something if you rush through one visit to get to the next. It may be worth contacting Mr Bloggs to inform him you are running late and to check his wellbeing. Think about what you say to him. Do not give the impression his health needs are low on your priority list.

You could also call back to base to inform colleagues of your situation. Someone may be able to cover on your behalf or slot in a later appointment with Mr Bloggs.

Make sure that your team always has a person on hand who can offer advice over the phone if you are unsure what to do. Your team leader would rather have four phone calls from you than another crisis to manage.

Increasing your skills

It is your duty as a nurse to constantly update your skills. The most useful way of doing this is by relating your ongoing training and professional development to your specialty. The RCN has a good network for specialties and publishes a journal for nearly all of them.

The NHS has developed a range of 'skills escalators' which are designed to help nurses and other health professionals advance their careers. You should discuss these with your line manager and ensure they are in place for your role.

Employers' obligations

Your employer is obliged to ensure that all staff have the opportunity to build on their skills. And as the watchwords in the NHS are 'recruitment and retention', any employer worth his or her salt will be keeping a close eye on this. They want to keep you working for them. You should receive regular updates from your employer on what training is available. But you should also keep an eye on the professional journals to ensure you have a good grasp on what is happening in nursing politically. For example, there is a drive to increase the number of nurses who can prescribe from an albeit limited list of drugs and dressings. And the role of 'modern matron' creates an opportunity for nurses to increase their skills and responsibilities without turning their backs on what they are good at – caring for patients (see pages 63–71 for an insight into being a modern matron in today's NHS).

Spotting opportunities

When it comes to increasing your skills, don't expect an invitation. Do some research into the opportunities for further training. The RCN and Unison, as trade unions and professional organizations, offer a wealth of advice.

Attending conferences is also a good means of networking with people working in your field and connecting with advances in your specialty. Conference places cost money, but your employer will probably have a budget for this. Keep an eye on the professional journals to see what is coming up and get your request in early. Keep pushing on the door. The worst thing that could happen is your employer will have to say no.

Further reading

Morris S, Willcocks G, Knasel E. *How to Lead a Winning Team.* London: Pearson Education, 2000.

Quick TL. *Successful Team Building.* New York: Amacom, 1992.

Results from the RCN membership surveys 2001/02. Commissioned by the Royal College of Nursing and conducted by Jane Ball and Geoff Pike from Employment Research (available from www.rcn.org.uk).

communicating clearly

Clear, concise and effective communication skills are essential for all nurses, from the most junior right up to the director of nursing. Nurses spend a lot of their time talking to patients and explaining procedures. They are generally regarded as being better at communicating than doctors!

> good communication depends not only on content but also delivery

To be a successful nurse, you must develop the ability to establish a relationship with patients, but also with colleagues, managers and other healthcare professionals. Good communication depends not only on content but also on delivery. Both need to be adjusted according to the audience and the setting in which you find yourself.

Talking to your patients

Talking to patients is not always easy, particularly on a busy clinic or ward. There are, however, a number of golden rules that, if followed, will help you to do this effectively.

When you first meet a patient introduce yourself by name, tell them your role and why you are here. Listen carefully to what the patient has to say and avoid interrupting. Establish eye contact and smile, if appropriate. Always take care to speak clearly and concisely. You should try to avoid jargon, abbreviations and acronyms, and technical terms. Give the patient opportunities to ask questions. Have stock phrases at the ready such as 'do you understand?' or 'is that OK?' Make it clear that it is fine to ask.

If you are about to perform a procedure, explain exactly what you are about to do. Warn the patient if it is going to be painful or uncomfortable. Important messages may need to be repeated and reinforced several times. Stressed and anxious patients may absorb only a fraction of what they are told. If possible, give your patient literature, a leaflet for example, that provides relevant and understandable information about his or her treatment and condition. Tell patients about websites and support groups, and make contact details available. Make it clear that you are focused and that you care. It may be helpful for the patient if you write down the key points about the treatment.

important messages

may need to

be repeated

Never give the impression that you are in a hurry, even though you usually are. Be especially patient with elderly patients and children. Talk directly to them, not to relatives or carers who may be present.

Breaking bad news

Many people believe only doctors and policemen get to break bad news, but nurses do it too, increasingly so as their roles expand and their responsibilities grow. Studies have shown that a growing number of patients want to know about and understand their diagnosis.

If a patient has a terminal illness they will usually be given this information by their doctor or consultant. But nurses will often have to follow on from this by imparting news if a procedure has failed. And patients will often speak to a nurse following a terminal diagnosis. Many patients have a deferential attitude to doctors and 'don't want to bother them'. They will often ask nurses to explain more fully what the doctor has told them, so the same techniques apply.

Nurses are much more involved in breaking bad news to relatives when a patient dies or his or her health deteriorates. Breaking bad news can be a harrowing experience. A relative whose mother has just died may experience incredible grief and need to be comforted. On the other hand, he or she may well feel very angry, lash out, or apportion blame.

The first thing you must do is to find somewhere quiet. Many hospitals have special rooms set aside for breaking bad news or to give relatives a place for some peace. Ask the relative to sit down. Say what you have to immediately. Don't prevaricate. State it simply and concisely. Speak clearly. Don't shout, but don't whisper either. The last thing you want is to have to repeat yourself. Show empathy – say that you are sorry. Some guidelines for breaking bad news are summarized in Table 4.

Table 4

Guidelines for breaking bad news

Preparation
- Familiarize yourself with all the information about the patient. If a patient has died, ensure you know the details of when and how
- Have the patient's notes with you so you can offer as much information as the relative needs

Talking to patients or relatives
- Ensure you have plenty of time to talk
- Offer patients or relatives time to be alone if they wish
- Avoid interruptions (bleeper, other colleagues)
- Explain the situation honestly and sensitively
- Use plain English
- Allow pauses for questions
- Be empathic and don't be afraid to say 'sorry' or 'I don't know'
- Encourage questions

It's a strange thing to say, but breaking bad news can be done very well and you may even feel good about how you did it afterwards. Done badly and the person will never forgive you. Done well, and they will never forget you.

Supporting partners and close relatives

The impact of an illness and its treatment on a patient's partner is an important, but often neglected, area. The treatments used in prostate cancer, for example, commonly affect sexual function and these need to be discussed not only with the patient, but also with his partner. The consequences of loss of libido, erectile dysfunction and ejaculatory disturbances must be explained sympathetically to both partners. Failure to do so effectively may have a devastatingly negative impact on people's relationships. Men, and older men in particular, diagnosed as suffering from cancer are particularly reliant on the social support that stems from intimate relationships, and withdrawal from sexual relationships may have severe consequences on both their quality of life and overall health.

In the case of a terminal illness, partners will experience a mixture of emotions. They feel sad for their partner. They will also fear living after their partner has gone. They may have worries about telling children. Really good nurses can pick up on these fears. Find out if you have a counselling service at your hospital. Put relatives in touch with support groups so they can talk to people in the same situation as them.

Communicating with dying patients

Death doesn't always come to us as a friend, and in no other situation is good communication between health professionals, patient and relatives more important, or potentially more fraught. Remember that, in a family, death is associated with all sorts of concomitant tensions. Not only are the relatives trying to deal with the demise of a loved one, but they may also have to confront other compromising issues, such as financial hardship, feelings of guilt and childcare issues.

"it is not so much the quantity of time, but the quality of time that is critical"

One problem of which we should be acutely aware is the lack of public understanding about the way today's NHS functions. Many people have fond memories of how things were years ago – plenty of beds and access to the same doctor continually. However, things have changed. The level of emergency admissions means that patients are placed where a bed is available, often on wards where staff are not experts in that patient's condition. This inevitably leads to fragmented communication. Advances in medicine mean there is a much greater reluctance to accept death as an inevitable outcome, no matter how old or how ill the patient.

The key to the problem is good communication. Lack of information makes people feel powerless, and powerlessness can lead to aggression. Timely and appropriate information must be given to the patient and relatives in a friendly, professional and sympathetic manner. In the words of Dame Cicely Saunders, founder of the hospice movement, "Remember, 5 minutes conversation on a timely basis can save hours of work later on.

It is not so much the quantity of time, but the quality of time that is critical."

Communicating with colleagues and managers

To be a successful nurse you have to be perceived as such by your colleagues and managers. If you want to climb the career ladder you need to start building your reputation as a knowledgeable practitioner who pulls his or her weight. You also need to be friendly and approachable. So start building your reputation now.

The way you communicate with colleagues on clinical matters is critical to the position in which they place you in their own mental hierarchy. It may seem blindingly obvious, but keep in mind that people prefer a friendly, affable, optimistic colleague to a taciturn, abrasive and pessimistic one, and are far more likely to relate to and support the former. Nurses work under enormous pressure. You will often feel tired. But everyone is in the same boat, and no one can bear a moaner.

Your professionalism speaks volumes about who you are. Try and stay out of any bitching and backbiting. If you share negative views about a colleague with another, they may well suspect you'd be equally scathing about them. Don't be afraid to talk to managers. They are under pressure to make the most of your skills and most of all to keep you working for them! Get to know who your managers are and what they do. Don't be deferential. When communicating with them be direct and honest. They will value you the more for it.

First impressions are particularly important. If you are in a new job, shaking hands, maintaining eye contact and remembering the name of a new colleague is helpful. Remember that every corridor meeting is a communication exercise. After meeting or talking to you, people will form an impression – good communication helps to make it a good impression.

Making presentations

You may dread it, but if you want to succeed as a nurse you're going to have to do it at some point in your career. There are dozens of great nurse presenters on the conference circuit and they are not all the great and the good. The best presentations are from people who have done something wonderful to improve patient care. And that is very often nurses who have patient contact every day of their lives. It's also your duty to share good practice.

it's your **duty** to share **good practice**

Good presentations do not just happen – they are the result of careful planning and preparation. Interesting and relevant content, clear delivery and a variety of visual and auditory techniques all contribute to an effective presentation.

Developing the text

The spoken word needs to be much simpler and more straightforward than the written word. To make your message clear, remember the adage: 'Tell them what you are going to tell them, tell them, and then tell them what you have told them.' Use plain, simple English and try to illustrate your points with word pictures; many people will remember information that is told as a story or anecdote rather than dry facts or ideas.

illustrate your **points** with **word pictures**

Know and connect with your audience. Ask yourself 'what is the audience hoping to get out of this talk?' At the same time, consider your message and how best to convey it. Make it clear very early on in the talk why your subject is relevant and exactly 'what's in it' for the attendees. Be clear about what you want the audience to take away with them.

It is crucial to be thoroughly prepared for your presentation.

- Research your topic and write one long draft – set out all your ideas and facts.
- Work through this draft and underline the key points.
- Write these out on separate pieces of paper, and then go back to your first draft and find statements, facts or examples that corroborate your main points. Use these sparingly. Your audience's time is precious – do not waste it with inappropriate, too detailed or irrelevant information.

- Use logical development and try to link one major point with the next. Mark the points that can be made more effectively with a slide or overhead.
- Stand back and ask yourself: is the message relevant and clear, and what will it give the audience?

Preparing your delivery

However well prepared your text, it will not be appreciated unless it is well delivered in a lively, enthusiastic fashion. Do not memorize your talk – you risk forgetting a segment and grinding to an embarrassing and seemingly eternal halt. If this happens at a major presentation you will blush at the memory for a very long time! Learn the first two lines of your talk and after that speak spontaneously. Write the key points on numbered cards. You will also have your slides or overheads as prompts, but get to know them intimately and avoid using them as a crutch by following them slavishly. Practise your talk four or five times. Do not just run through it silently – actually try to recreate the setting and speak your words out loud. Get a critical friend to listen to it. Time it. It should be neither too short nor too long.

> you never have a second chance to make a first impression

On the day, arrive early and check the facilities, such as slide-changing buttons, carefully before you ascend the podium. Think 'if it can go wrong, it will go wrong' and be prepared for emergencies. Finally, look after your own equipment carefully and treat your computer leads as a sailor would his ropes!

Making your presentation

Remember, you never have a second chance to make a first impression, so how you look is fundamental. Smart clothing will project the correct image. You should also appear confident and professional, but remain calm and relaxed throughout the proceedings.

After your talk, people will leave not only with the information that you have supplied (if they have listened), but also with an impression of you. This stems not from what you say, but how you say it (see Table 5). Body language – your posture, stance and arm movements – is an important part of your image.

Avoid the monotonous delivery that sedates an audience so effectively! Smile and enthuse – if you are not interested in your subject, why should your audience be? Use voice inflection, pauses, tone and pace – speak slowly, loudly and deliberately. Do not talk to your slides as you will inevitably turn away from the audience and the microphone. Humour is a powerful way to establish and maintain audience rapport. But making people laugh is not a matter of telling jokes. In general, avoid jokes unless you can deliver them with timing and congruence – a joke that falls flat stays down a long time, along with your talk! 'Fun' is not the same as 'funny'; often all you need to do to raise a smile and get the audience on your side is point out the odd or unusual aspects of something quite mundane.

Table 5

How to deliver your presentation effectively

- Dress comfortably and appropriately
- Try to stand squarely towards the audience, with legs slightly apart
- Make eye contact and remember not to ignore any section of the audience
- Have an arresting opening
- Use appropriate hand gestures
- Do not talk to your slides
- Speak slowly and inflect your voice
- Pause for emphasis, but speak in complete sentences
- Repeat important points
- Use concrete and specific examples
- Convey enthusiasm
- Pose questions and give possible answers
- Explain the significance of points
- Summarize the talk
- Suggest what the audience should do with the information

Most importantly, stick to the time limit you've been given. Running over time is very unprofessional and will have an impact on the time available for the next speaker.

Visual aids

Good slides or overheads will add interest to your presentation and provide another medium for communicating your key messages. They allow an audience to focus on the salient points. However, unclear, cluttered slides with spelling mistakes will do little to enhance your image and credibility. Follow the golden rules for effective visuals (Table 6) – 80% of what your audience remembers is what they see. Always check the size of the room that you will be presenting in.

Ensure that people at the back of the room will be able to read your slides, otherwise you risk losing their attention. Do not try to present too many slides – allow each slide to be shown long enough for everyone to read. As a guideline, a 15-minute presentation should be accompanied by no more than 15 slides. As each slide comes up, pause and then tell the audience what it says and what it means. Don't just read it out. They can do that themselves. This technique is known as 'clearing the visual'.

do not present too many slides

PowerPoint

Using PowerPoint to create a slide show for a presentation is becoming increasingly popular. In fact, everyone seems to be doing it! The reason for this is that it is a remarkably simple software program to work with.

Be careful if you do use it as computers have an annoying habit of going wrong at the crucial moment. It is always a good idea to back up a PowerPoint presentation by making good old acetates of what you had hoped to present electronically.

Taking questions

Hopefully you will have a chairperson to manage this for you. A good chair will give you a little breather by saying something nice about you

Table 6

Making the most of slides and overheads

- Each slide or overhead should have a specific purpose; limit each to one main idea
- Be accurate – mistakes on visuals stand out like a sore thumb, forcing the speaker into apologetic mode
- Aim for simplicity and conciseness – do not overload your slide with information your audience doesn't have time to read
- Design slides so that the back row of your audience can see and understand them – if your slide is readable without any magnification when held up to a light, it should be effective when projected
- Use strong, bold sans serif typefaces (such as arial); don't use all capitals, lower case letters are more legible
- Use ample spacing between lines, no more than seven words per line and a maximum of seven lines per slide
- Ensure axes and data lines on graphs are sufficiently bold to be clearly visible
- Avoid punctuation; use bullet points
- Use light-coloured text (ideally yellow or white) on a dark background
- Use a consistent style between slides – slides can then be mixed and matched for future presentations
- Summarize the 'take-home' messages on your final slide

while you catch your breath and will have a question ready for you if all around are silent.

Leave a minimum of 10 minutes for questions. Try and think what issues might crop up or need clarifying.

Keep back a few pieces of information you could give when taking questions. This is a very impressive thing to do as it shows that you are enthusiastic, knowledgeable and thorough. Most audiences are friendly – they've willingly come to hear you. So relax in the knowledge that most are not there to catch you out.

Writing skills

Some people are naturally good writers. However, writing is a skill that can be improved by practice. Good writing comes from good planning and meticulous attention to detail (there are some tips in Table 7). Opportunities to write something come from two fronts. You may be commissioned to do something, or you may have an idea that you would like to pitch to an editor.

There is a very wide range of nursing journals that need to be fed good clinical material written by nurses. There are very general journals such as *Nursing Times* and *Nursing Standard*, but there are many specialist journals too. The RCN publishes lots of them.

If you are commissioned to write an article, it is probably because that editor has found out that you are an expert in your field, you have conducted some original research or you are doing something new that would be good to share with other nurses. Editors don't expect nurses to

Table 7
Tips for effective writing

- Try to explain what you mean in as few words as possible – most of what we write is far too verbose
- Use short words rather than long ones when you can
- Use jargon, abbreviations and acronyms only when writing exclusively for fellow specialists
- Restrict sentences to 15–20 words; aim to introduce only one 'idea' per sentence or clause
- Use bullet points to avoid hiding lengthy lists in your text (they help to break up text and make it less visually daunting)
- Use different levels of headings (having checked the style of the publication, of course) – these also help to break up the text
- Avoid clichés like the plague(!)
- Make sure that any figures are correct (especially drug doses) and that any statistics are accurate
- Keep your reader and your message in mind at all times

be award-winning writers. They are willing to do quite a bit of work on your original paper before publication. You will probably be sent guidelines as to what the editor wants. Examine them and look at examples of work in the journal in question.

If you want to pitch an idea, have a look at the various journals and think which one your idea would most appeal to. Ask yourself, 'who is the reader?' Keep the reader in mind throughout the writing process.

Many nurses write articles and send them directly to the journal. But it's much better if you call the journal and discuss your idea with the appropriate member of staff. They will tell you whether or not your idea is on the right track and will give you some guidance on how to write it. This means when it reaches the right desk it is more likely to be recognized and read.

ask yourself, 'who is the reader?'

Research your topic thoroughly and put all your ideas, supporting facts and arguments down on paper. Start by drafting an outline. You need a beginning, a middle and an end. Draw some conclusions.

Organize your main points in order of importance, adding details to support each main point. At this stage, you are ready to write. Stick to the outline and start with the main ideas and their supporting details. Once this is done, revise the text and consider how well your message has been conveyed and whether the reader will be satisfied.

Submitting to a journal

If you are submitting a paper to a peer-reviewed journal and your work is not rejected at the first hurdle, you will have to respond to the reviewers' comments and may have to do a bit of rewriting. You will also be expected to check page proofs. Read your work through carefully before submission – pay particular attention to drug regimens and dosages, experimental data and the results of any calculations. Also, double check the results of any other studies that you refer to.

Follow the instructions for submission of articles carefully and always keep copies of everything that you send to the journal.

There is more advice on publishing your work on pages 143–153.

Working on a sponsored publication

Writing for a pharmaceutical company-sponsored publication can be both lucrative and satisfying. It's a current trend for pharma companies to produce very professional one-off publications as it is more subtle than advertising and allows them to demonstrate that they are interested in patient care, not just profits.

More and more nurses are getting involved in this area, especially in the infection control and wound care specialties as they are very product-based. These publications are usually of the highest quality and it can be a thrill to see your name adorning such an attractive piece of work.

You may be approached by either a product manager or other representative from a pharmaceutical company, or by an account manager or editor working on the pharmaceutical company's behalf. Before committing yourself to anything, you must make sure that you are completely clear about your role, the aim of the publication, how your name will be used, who has editorial control, how much work is involved and the schedule. The type of project varies widely, but each and every publication has a role in marketing the company's drug or product. Make sure you are comfortable with that.

Further reading

Albert T. *Medical Journalism: The Writer's Guide.* Oxford: Radcliffe Medical Press, 1992.

Albert T. *Winning the Publications Game: How to Get Published Without Neglecting Your Patients.* Oxford: Radcliffe Medical Press, 1996.

Barker A. *Improve Your Communication Skills.* London: Kogan Page, 2000.

managing crises

Although crises in the health service are much more common than in the airline business, airline personnel receive far more training in crisis management than nurses do. Learning to cope with and learn from crises is now an essential skill for a successful nurse. Litigation is becoming increasingly common in the NHS, and indeed throughout the world. One reason for this is undoubtedly poor-quality interpersonal working relationships. Another is that patients have come to expect much more from health professionals. Many are better informed about their health and the treatment they can expect from the NHS. They are therefore less submissive and more critical.

Besides clinical ability, there are a number of key components of good clinical practice.

- You should practise sound clinical management. This is not only about clinical ability, but means sticking to your own area of expertise and avoiding the temptation to cut corners.
- Competent administration is integral to good clinical practice. Get organized.
- Clear communication is essential, including the keeping of accurate, up-to-date records.
- Apart from being clinically competent, a good nurse must be able to break bad news, provide counselling, obtain consent from patients for any form of intervention and generally deal kindly, professionally and effectively with people.

You are responsible and accountable for your own actions. Nurses are often the first point of contact for patients and relatives when they come into a care setting. So it's a relief that good clinical practice and effective interpersonal skills will avert most crises – all you have to do is make sure you have these qualities in your arsenal.

> you are responsible and accountable for your own actions

When dealing with a crisis, the most important rule is to put a human face on the problem. Try to deal with it quickly without passing the buck if you can avoid it. When a crisis occurs which involves a patient, the situation demands sympathy, understanding and, when a mistake has been made, an apology. Importantly, an expression of regret ('I'm terribly sorry this has happened') is not an admission of guilt.

It is equally important to deal with the individual's perceptions ('I can see how this must seem to you') and not just the facts. Finally, you should remain polite, honest, caring, professional and dignified at all times. Responding aggressively and defensively ('it's not my fault') is a very destructive way of dealing with a bad situation. It is also vital for your colleagues, who could find themselves in a similar situation, to learn from the mistake.

The possibility that an adverse event has arisen because of a more fundamental problem should always be considered. This is the essence of 'risk management'. By monitoring and learning from all unusual, unintentional or adverse events and looking for patterns in their occurrence, potential crises may be averted. Only when effective risk management exists will you and those around you be assured that any crisis is a one in a million occurrence in an otherwise excellent track record. People may come and go but a safety culture must prevail. Trusts should have protocols for dealing with all kinds of bad situations, from aggression to serious medical and clinical errors. Every time you join a new team or enter a new working environment you should ask to see these protocols. This is not paranoia. It's common sense and you need to be prepared for any eventuality.

you need to be prepared for any eventuality

Coping with violence

Much has been written on the issue of violence against healthcare workers, most notably nurses. Over 95 000 incidents of violence and aggression were reported in the NHS across the UK in 2001–02, a 13% rise on the previous year. The RCN 2002 Membership Survey found that around one in three nurses had been physically assaulted during their careers. More than a half of all nurses working in mental health and learning disabilities, and 45% of those in adult general nursing were harassed or assaulted by patients in the 12 months prior to the survey.

Nurses working nights are more exposed to harassment than others. More than half of male nurses were harassed or assaulted by patients in the 12 months period prior to the survey compared with 38% of women – but remember, the nursing workforce is around 94% female. The high number of men being assaulted is related to a concentration of male nurses in fields where harassment is more prevalent, notably mental health.

With nurses facing so much aggression and threatening behaviour every day, it is surprising to find that fewer than one in 20 nurses responding to a *Nursing Times* survey in 2002 said they had received support from the NHS in pressing charges when attacked and only one in ten were offered counselling after they were attacked.

Why it happens

Why is there so much violence in the NHS? Quite simply, while the NHS has improved immensely over the past decade, demand still outweighs supply. Nurses are often too busy to explain things properly to patients. Patients are passed from pillar to post in what is possibly the biggest bureaucracy in the country. When people are ill emotions run high.

Patients and their relatives often lash out in the healthcare setting because they are frustrated (after a 4-hour wait in A&E for example), are not fully informed of their

> when people are ill emotions run high

prognosis or are drunk or under the influence of drugs. As nurses are often the first point of contact for patients, especially in A&E, they are usually first on the receiving end of any attack. Also, as about 94% of people reading this will be women and most of the perpetrators of violence are men, your assailant is confident he is less likely to end up worse off.

It is unacceptable that people who spend their lives caring for others should face the daily threat of verbal or physical assault. Violent and abusive behaviour should not be, and on the whole is not, tolerated in the NHS. No one has the right to abuse or harass you. Violent assault is a crime, and should be treated as such.

Measures that can be taken

A lot has been done over the years in the health service to protect nurses and other colleagues from violent attack. The government's 'zero tolerance campaign', launched in 2001, gave the NHS the go-ahead to deny patients treatment if they attack NHS staff. National guidelines support NHS trusts to draw up their own policies on withdrawing treatment from patients whose behaviour is unacceptable – verbal abuse, threats, violence, drug or alcohol abuse in hospital, and destruction of property. The exception to the rule is mental health patients, who are exempt from having treatment withdrawn. The zero tolerance campaign and national guidelines encourage trusts to develop local policies on withholding treatment from violent and abusive patients. The guidelines suggest patients should be offered a verbal warning and a written warning before treatment is withheld. In exceptional circumstances – where there's a threat of serious and imminent danger or a serious incident is taking or has taken place – treatment can be immediately withheld. Treatment may be withdrawn for a limited period of no more than 12 months – and only as a last resort measure.

This is obviously flawed, and assumes that all patients who are violent are known to the organization which is treating them. This is not always the case. A large proportion of violence occurs in A&E, where patients have perhaps dropped in for the first time. The violence may happen before the nurses even have their names.

A National Audit Office report in 2003 examined the extent and impact of violence and aggression within the NHS, and evaluated the effectiveness of the actions taken by the Department of Health and the NHS trusts to combat these problems. The report identifies nurses and other NHS staff who have direct interaction with the public – for example, ambulance and A&E staff, and staff who work in acute mental health units – as having a higher risk of exposure to violence and aggression. The Audit Office suggests that attempts to combat these problems since 2000 have largely failed. Indeed, a number of research projects have demonstrated clear links between violence and aggression and staff sickness absence, turnover and lost productivity.

The Audit Office says that while all NHS trusts "have embraced the values set out in the campaign", they have not always turned words into action.

- Many trusts fail to provide staff with the training needed to deal with violence and aggression.

- Many trusts fail to offer counselling to those members of staff who have been attacked.
- Many trusts fail to pursue criminal prosecutions or to support staff wishing to pursue civil actions.
- Security measures vary across trusts.

The Audit Office also suggests that often members of staff do not report violent incidents against them because they fear that this may be viewed as a reflection of their own inability to manage difficult situations. Staff also believe that no action will be taken or that the NHS trust is unlikely to give them adequate support.

What you can do

Work has been stepped up to eradicate violence from the healthcare setting, but the problems do not seem to want to disappear. So we have to manage it. From 2004, as part of their accreditation process, security specialists in health bodies have been receiving training in law-enforcement techniques, such as interviewing and taking statements from witnesses.

While the problem is clearly a big one, thankfully most day-to-day violence encountered in the healthcare setting is verbal or threatened rather than physical. A dissatisfied patient may occasionally be verbally abusive, and it is important to help to prevent the situation escalating. The presence of a third independent person, if only to corroborate your version of events at a subsequent enquiry, is important. If you are unsure how to respond to a verbally abusive patient, relative or even a member of staff, it is best to say nothing as any response might fuel their anger. Faced with silence, most people eventually run out of steam and begin to feel foolish.

if you are unsure how to respond it is best to say nothing

Never touch an abusive person as any form of body contact may be construed as assault, however well-meaning your intention. Nevertheless, your duty does not extend to having to tolerate abuse of any kind. If an attempt at reasonable discussion fails, then quietly, politely, but firmly terminate the interview as soon as possible, document the occurrence carefully and inform the risk manager for the hospital trust of the events, ideally with corroboration from an independent witness. In the case of an abusive patient, notify the person's GP, if known, of events.

Real physical violence in hospitals is comparatively rare, at least in Western Europe. Threatened physical violence by angry patients or by patients who are under the influence of drugs or alcohol is much more common – but this can be frightening all the same. If necessary, the patient can be physically removed from the hospital. Never become physically threatening yourself – this only makes the situation worse. If the patient needs to be restrained, always involve hospital security staff or the police as they are trained in the proper techniques. All hospitals now have 'risk managers' and security staff to deal with such situations.

Training

There is now a range of training in the recognition, prevention and management of violence and aggression and conflict resolution which nurses can access. Most good trusts, having responded to government guidelines, will supply that training, especially to staff working in high-risk areas such as A&E and mental health.

Working with difficult colleagues

You can choose your friends, but you can't choose your blood relatives or colleagues. Many so-called 'difficult colleagues' are simply people you would not choose to associate with socially. Nonetheless, they may have their own circle of professional friends who would view you similarly. On the other hand, many healthcare environments have a 'difficult' employee who seems to be a law unto him or herself. Such people usually continue to act in this way because no one has ever discussed with them the fact that their behaviour might be considered inappropriate – assuming that they are indeed a cause for concern. Reasons for talking to a colleague about their conduct include:
- how they talk to patients and colleagues
- problems associated with drug and alcohol consumption
- actions that affect the health and safety of others
- behaviour that may be offensive or embarrassing to others.

Some people are unaware of the effect their behaviour has on others. When they find out, they might be upset and try to change, or they might become abusive or aggressive. Usually, the best course of action is to confront the individual, bring your concerns to their attention and then attempt to address the issues. Attempting to resolve such a situation with a sympathetic discussion is highly preferable to allowing it to escalate. It is a question of being assertive rather than aggressive. Although such a discussion may potentially be unpleasant, if conducted politely and in an even-handed manner, it is often productive.

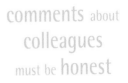

comments about colleagues must be honest

If a colleague's behaviour continues to be a problem, then you should inform the appropriate person, such as the nurse director or human resources director of your trust. This is particularly important if you suspect substance abuse, or anything else that could be potentially harmful, to be a factor.

Your comments about colleagues must be honest. People will resent you if you exaggerate a difficult colleague's behaviour just because you don't happen to like them. Equally, you should never play down bad behaviour in a colleague you happen to like. The safety of patients must be your priority at all times. Your primary duty is to your patients and other colleagues for any such professional breach of conduct at work. So being objective is very important.

Dealing with sexual harassment

One person may feel that certain behaviour constitutes sexual harassment while another individual may consider the same 'a piece of harmless fun'. Nurses, unfortunately, are often stereotyped as 'goers', sexually promiscuous, coquettish. Look at how nurses are, and have been, portrayed in the media. Carry On's Barbara Windsor nurse character still haunts the nursing profession. Male nurses are stereotyped too. At grassroots level they are thin on the ground and often victimized for doing 'women's work'.

Sexual harassment comes in many guises. Many victims of sexual harassment tolerate it, mainly because they barely notice it. They may even find it amusing in small doses, and laugh about it. However, it is never a good idea to tolerate such behaviour.

As a nurse you should be vigilant about sexual harassment. This is what you can do if someone speaks or acts inappropriately towards you.

- Tell them that you are uncomfortable with this behaviour – that it offends you or scares you.
- Take yourself out of the situation – if an individual seems to be targeting you inappropriately, ensure that you are never alone with this person.
- Give no encouragement. If someone is hassling you, don't respond to them. Do not engage in friendly banter. This person will degrade you in some way, although this may not necessarily be their intention.
- If a patient touches you inappropriately, challenge them immediately, in a loud voice for other people to hear.
- Keep things out in the open. Confide in a colleague if you think someone is harassing you, even if it is only minor pestering.

If things escalate, report the offender to a third party who can take independent action. Such action might be simply to draw the matter to the attention of the wrongdoer who may then stop their inappropriate behaviour. Indeed, some people are horrified to find that they are perceived in this way when they genuinely felt they were being 'friendly and amusing'.

More serious cases should always be dealt with by a nursing or medical director. Offenders should be reminded that it is not what they meant to say or do but how others perceived it that is important.

keep things
out in the open

Dealing with discrimination

As everybody knows, racial and sexual discrimination are illegal. Although the law sets the standards by which we are expected to live, we are all aware that, in practice, these are regularly breached.

Irrespective of racial or gender issues, favouritism has always existed. In our dealings with others, we should try to be fair as we would not wish to be subject to such bias ourselves. Nowadays, anybody who is involved in interview processes is obliged to take a course in which matters of racial and sexual discrimination are addressed. Participants will be 'trained' not to discriminate against applicants on the grounds of race, sex, religion, or sexuality. Application forms are being designed increasingly to exclude discrimination so far as is possible.

The government is committed to promoting diversity in the NHS. It is one of the main tenets of the NHS Plan of 2000. Positively Diverse is a national organizational development programme which aims to change the culture of NHS organizations. International recruitment is a hot potato, with many nurses arriving here from all over the world. Many do not speak good English, which leaves them wide open to discrimination. Positively Diverse has been developed to address equality and diversity issues based on understanding how staff feel.

What you should do

As with violence, the NHS is aware that discrimination is a problem. Some patients, especially older ones, simply refuse to be cared for by a black nurse. But, as with violence, your trust should have a policy on promoting diversity. A good nurse is a good nurse, and patients need to be pulled into line with sustainable behavioural policies.

If you do face discrimination:

- tell your line manager
- challenge offensive remarks and behaviour, especially from colleagues and from patients and relatives
- support colleagues who are being discriminated against
- contact your trade union or professional organization and seek their advice
- blow the whistle on institutional discrimination in whatever form.

Handling journalists

Dealing with the media is an increasingly important communication skill for health professionals. Trusts often send senior staff on media training, but let's be honest – if you are just starting out in nursing you are unlikely to be called to comment on behalf of the trust!

You may well be approached by a journalist when something negative happens in your area of work. Discover what your employer's policy is on dealing with the media. Most trusts these days have a press and communications function and most will have a policy where journalists will always be directed to the press or communications officer if they have any questions or wish to speak to someone on an issue. However, healthcare is full of great human interest stories.

discover your **employer's policy** on **dealing** with the **media**

A good journalist wants the view from the frontline staff and may just cold-call your unit. You may answer the phone and before you know it, you are deep in a conversation you didn't mean to have. So watch out. This could land you in trouble.

Most managers in the health service are fairly cynical about the media, probably because they only seem to be interested in negative stories about bad care and dirty hospitals. But there are more good things than bad going on in hospitals today and it is frontline staff like you who know about them. Tell your managers and tell your press office. You may get the opportunity to talk to journalists about something you are proud of.

Disasters do happen in the healthcare setting – and don't the media love it when they do. As grassroots practitioners, nurses are a journalist's dream when reporting on a crisis. But, unfortunately, nurses rarely get the chance to speak out. Communications directors and corporate communication strategies make it increasingly difficult for journalists to access practitioners at the coalface of the NHS.

It only takes one unfortunate incident to spark a frenzy of antagonistic media interest, destroying staff commitment that has been built up over many years, literally overnight. If such a situation arises, it is essential that your line manager establishes the facts surrounding the case and obtains group support. Everyone involved in the incident should meet to develop a common understanding of what exactly has taken place and how it should be handled. It is vital for everyone to have clear and concise facts at their fingertips. As a nurse you may be excluded from talking to the press about a crisis, but you still have to communicate with colleagues and patients around you who could be affected by adverse publicity.

Staying in control

Most trusts have a designated press officer to deal with journalists. Elicit their support early on. Never attempt to go it alone. Be very wary about unsolicited telephone calls from journalists. Before answering their questions, try to find out what they know, where they got their information from and what their slant is. If you do speak to journalists, always begin by giving some sound, positive information about your area of work, thus providing evidence that the unit normally works well and effectively. Use other authoritative sources, such as Royal Colleges and specialist associations, to corroborate your position, if you can. If you do not seize the opportunity to put good, positive news about clinical practice into the

better to be honest than look stupid

public domain, the public will only ever hear the bad news, and all the good work that we do will be discounted. Above all, if you don't know the answer to a question, say so. Don't wing it. Better to be honest than look stupid.

If you do get the opportunity to tell your story, it's a good idea to get the journalist to tell you in advance the kind of questions they'd like to ask you. Keep your answers simple, short and straightforward. Before the interview, try to think of a catchy 'sound bite' that encapsulates your message, and end the interview on an upbeat and positive note.

Beware of making an impromptu remark that may be taken out of context. Above all, avoid breaching patient confidentiality or denigrating your colleagues publicly.

Before accepting a call from a journalist, think carefully about what you want to say and try to put a positive spin on the issue in question. Table 8 has some general guidelines for talking to journalists.

Table 8

Simple guidelines for talking to journalists

- If you are cold-called by a journalist, ask them to explain exactly what they want to talk about. What are they writing – a news story or a feature? If you are not quite sure what to say, or feel you would like to gather your thoughts, ask if you can call them back
- If possible, find a room where you can talk privately. If you are nervous, the last thing you want is your colleagues listening in or interruptions to put you off your flow
- Think about the point you want to get over. The journalist wants you to say something interesting or enlightening. Write down what you want to say. Be concise and punchy. "Just compare the funds to develop chief executives with money for nurse leadership. The maths tells its own story" is a great comment. Compare it with "there's not enough funding for nurse leaders". Which would you like to have said?
- When you have made your point, stop talking. Let the journalist do the work
- If you have figures and statistics, offer them
- If you do not feel able to answer a question, say so. You will feel more stupid if you talk rubbish than if you just say, "I don't know"
- Ask when the article will be published. Tell your manager or anyone else who needs to know

Further reading

The guidance on zero tolerance is available at www.nhs.uk/zerotolerance.

National Audit Office. *A Safer Place to Work: Protecting NHS Hospital and Ambulance Staff from Violence and Aggression.* London: TSO, 2003 (available from www.nao.org.uk/publications/nao_reports/02-03/0203527.pdf).

career destinations

"trust one who has gone through it"
Virgil, *The Aeneid*
Roman epic poet (70 BC–19 BC)

Nurse consultant

Clare Abley, Nurse Consultant – Vulnerable Older Adults, Newcastle, North Tyneside and Northumberland Mental Health NHS Trust

Nurse consultant posts were introduced by the government in 2000 in an attempt to provide a career path for senior nurses who wanted to stay in clinical practice. At the time, recruitment and retention of nurses was high on the government agenda and these posts were seen as a 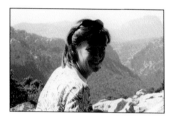 way of holding on to skilled and experienced nurses who might have otherwise left the NHS. All posts have the same core components of expert practice, education, training and development, service and practice development and research, audit and evaluation. The role does not include operational management, but change management, project management and strategic management are all essential aspects of the job.

A nurse consultant post may appeal to you if you enjoy a challenge, are self-motivated and, most importantly, wish to remain in clinical practice whilst influencing strategic development. The first nurse consultants were trailblazers. But a yearning to be at the forefront of developments to the nursing profession is now less important, with posts being viewed increasingly as a core component of high-quality service provision.

The role

Nurse consultant posts vary according to specialty and also according to the requirements of individual trusts. Some posts have a predetermined and clearly defined clinical component, such as running a particular clinic or managing a case load, whereas others allow the postholder to develop his or her own clinical role. Generally, the clinical roles undertaken by nurse consultants are outside the boundaries of traditional clinical nursing practice, either involving tasks that were previously carried out by doctors, such as performing endoscopies, or providing a new service in response to the changing needs of healthcare. The scope of expert practice is wide and also includes developing the practice of other nurses and multidisciplinary teams. This may be done locally or nationally.

the scope of expert practice is wide

Working as a nurse consultant, although challenging at times (particularly when establishing a new post), is very rewarding. You have the opportunity to identify what needs to be done to improve things for patients and to make the necessary changes in the way that you think best fits the situation. One such improvement might be to the care of patients with dementia on acute medical wards. You may have spent time in a particular clinical area and have used your professional judgment to identify the need for improvement, or you might be responding to feedback from carers. Or you may have been asked by the director of nursing to consider how the finding of a national report on this topic might be implemented in the trust.

At a local level, your initiative might include:

- setting up and leading a steering group
- empowering staff to make changes
- delivering or providing training for staff
- setting standards for practice or searching the literature to find ones that already exist
- carrying out an audit of practice or supporting others to do so
- possibly working in the clinical area as an expert role model or undertaking research into this aspect of care.

In carrying out this work you will also have to motivate others if you are to be successful in achieving sustainable change.

Highs and lows

Every job has its highs and lows and many nurse consultants who are new in the post describe their experiences in the early days as swinging from one extreme to the other – one day experiencing a great sense of achievement and the next extreme frustration or low morale. Most settle into their roles and experience rapid and extensive personal development. Those who decide the job is not for them use it as a stepping stone to a different type of role. One thing's for sure, though – you will never be bored in your work as a nurse consultant.

Setting your own agenda

The autonomy afforded by the role is great if you are self-directed and capable of identifying what needs to be done and mustering the resources (personal and material) to have a real impact. If you need more direction, you might feel somewhat 'at sea' and that those in authority are not providing you with the necessary support. Often those in authority are as unsure about the role and what it can achieve as you are, so there is a real need to set your own agenda and deliver, making sure, of course, that you communicate what you are doing. With time you will develop 'a following' who will support you and drive forward your ideas. You will now be able to relax a little and enjoy the job, knowing that you are not the only one who is striving to achieve your goals. You should also make time to celebrate the success of those working with you, which will help you to recharge your batteries before moving on to your next challenge! You will experience a huge sense of pride and a real buzz as you witness personal development and achievement in your nursing colleagues.

> with **time** you will
> develop 'a following'

Developing the role

As a nurse consultant you will be expected to shape the future development of your own role. You may also have the chance to shape new roles, perhaps by being asked to comment on job descriptions, and to influence the development of new nurse consultant posts. Funding for posts is a real issue, however, so your case for a new post must be convincing and the added value demonstrable. As more posts are created, there is the opportunity to have a combined voice as a group of experienced and senior clinicians working within a particular specialty and thus achieve greater influence nationally and even internationally.

Being effective

The possibilities for improving care for patients are endless, but you have to learn to take on what is achievable and not try to do everything. At times the role can be overwhelming in its scope, so having a focus, sharing the load by involving others and constantly questioning whether this is something that really has to be taken on by you as a nurse consultant (as opposed to someone else), are all highly important if you are to be effective. Another trap to avoid is taking on work that you simply enjoy, regardless of whether it is really your job to do it.

Balancing proactivity and reactivity

The modernization of the health service continues at a rapid and often frenetic pace. This provides an ideal climate for introducing new initiatives and, as a nurse consultant, you can ensure that these focus on improving patient care and are not done in a piecemeal fashion that merely pays lip service to government policy. However, the strategic nature of the role also supports working in a less reactive and more proactive way, developing a vision for the future and pre-empting problems before they arise. Most people have a natural tendency to be either reactive or proactive. As a nurse consultant, you will have the opportunity to achieve a balance between these two approaches and to encourage others to do so.

take on what is achievable

The rewards

As a nurse consultant you have the opportunity to set the direction for the future of nursing within your specialty, for nursing as a whole and for healthcare in general. This doesn't mean that you will have sole responsibility for delivering that vision, although sometimes it feels as if you have! As a 'big picture', this may seem overwhelming, but the personal rewards of being asked to contribute to a briefing paper for the chief nursing officer, delivering an inspiring presentation at the trust nursing conference, being asked to sit on a national group reviewing policy in a certain area or seeing your article in print are self-evident. Few nurse consultants take up their post being able to influence at a national level, but those who are successful will have developed a diverse range of skills and will know when to use them to best effect.

Comparing the clinical nurse specialist role

Although certain aspects of the clinical nurse specialist and nurse consultant roles are similar (i.e. both involve clinical practice, education and practice development), nurse consultant posts generally occupy more senior positions within organizations – the expectation being that postholders will not only influence but also initiate and drive major changes in service delivery. Nurse consultants are usually directly accountable to the trust's executive director of nursing and play an active part in the development of nursing and healthcare in general, across organizations and nationally. From the perspective of the individual postholder, day-to-day autonomy is greater for nurse consultants and there is greater responsibility for creative problem-solving in complex and often risky situations.

If you want to be a nurse consultant

Training requirements

The training requirements for being a nurse consultant are not fixed, but you have to have a nursing qualification relevant to the post. For instance, if you want to be a nurse consultant working with adults, you need a registered general nurse (RGN) qualification, and if you want to work within mental health, you need a registered mental nurse (RMN) qualification. As with other qualified nursing posts, all nurse consultants must be registered with the Nursing and Midwifery Council (NMC). Most employers will also require applicants to have a degree and, in the majority of cases, a higher degree such as a masters or a PhD. Few stipulate that a PhD must be held before applying for the post, the willingness to undertake study at this level being seen as more important. A significant amount of experience within the specialty is also necessary in order to have credibility and to be able to do the job.

Personal qualities

No one nurse consultant will have all the qualities and skills that might be found in the archetypal postholder – concentrate your efforts on work that maximizes the use of your innate qualities, but try also to develop skills in areas that you find more difficult. Important personal qualities for the role include:

- self-assurance
- confidence
- determination and perseverance
- credibility
- authoritativeness (in a respectful way)
- a genuine commitment to improving the patient's experience and to working in partnership with others
- being able to come up with realistic but creative solutions
- sound professional judgment
- emotional intelligence.

Personal development

Many of the qualities and skills needed to be a successful nurse consultant can be developed over time as long as you have the motivation to succeed. There are numerous courses and development programmes available to staff within the NHS. Some develop self-awareness and others focus on knowledge acquisition or skill development. Being able to identify high-quality development opportunities that will help you to be more effective in your role is crucial. You will need to pursue ongoing development as the nature of the role changes in response to the current healthcare climate and as you take on new and exciting challenges. It is also wise to enlist the help and support of a mentor or supervisor who will give his or her view of your development needs.

- Decide on your priorities and focus on them
- Be proactive and take the initiative
- Before meetings, decide what you want to achieve and make sure you do!
- Always ask a carefully worded question or make a pertinent comment at conferences, open forums and group meetings
- Remember that people will not know what you are thinking unless you tell them
- Make deliberate decisions about what you say – do not let your emotions get in the way, and think about the message that you want to convey
- Remember why you became a nurse and never forget the patient
- Choose a good mentor whom you can trust
- Deal with your emotions; when necessary experience a healthy sense of detachment
- Deal with problems, do not let them 'fester'; thinking about a problem is often worse than solving it
- Don't waste time – sending a lengthy email when a quick phone call will do instead is wasting time!
- Produce work to a standard that is just above what is required – it's often a waste of time to produce a perfect piece of work, as your idea of perfect will be different from another's
- If you are unsure about what to do, always choose an option that is morally and ethically acceptable and fits with your own personal values – this will help to achieve peace of mind and respect from your colleagues
- Take your own advice – what advice would you give a colleague in a similar situation?
- Remember – you are the leader... but it is OK to lead from behind!
- Make time to recharge your batteries and strive to achieve a work/life balance

clinical nurse specialist

Angie Perrin, Senior Nurse/Clinical Nurse
Specialist, Stoma/Colorectal Nursing,
John Radcliffe Hospital, Oxford

The clinical nurse specialist (CNS) is viewed by most as an advanced nursing role. Most CNSs will have reached a level of experience before deciding to specialize. Specialist practice requires a wealth of experience, a sound knowledge base and a general experience of life. Some CNSs are taking on extended roles that were previously seen as more medical duties – those more traditionally carried out by doctors: for example, carrying out a flexible sigmoidoscopy or inserting a central line.

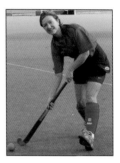

Establishing the role

The catalyst to the change was the publication of *The Scope of Professional Practice* by the United Kingdom Central Council for Nursing, Midwifery and Health Visiting (UKCC) in 1992. This encouraged nurses to extend and expand their roles. It was this paper, together with reports from the Department of Health highlighting that nurses should be working together with junior doctors to develop partnerships to deliver clinical care and reduce junior doctors' hours, that consequently gave nurses a little more rein to take on more responsibilities and further extend their roles. As a result, CNSs began to undertake specific activities that had traditionally been seen as medical and bring into them the art of nursing. This change in role is controversial for some, but it often allows patients to be seen more quickly in an already tightly stretched NHS, without compromising patient care. It is alleged anecdotally that seeing an experienced, skilful and knowledgeable nurse specialist is often perceived as being beneficial than seeing a more junior doctor with minimal experience.

Today, there are CNS positions in a countless number of specialties: for example, stoma care, diabetes, nutrition, and tissue viability.

Being a successful CNS

In my opinion, any good nurse is a successful nurse! But what makes a good nurse? Possessing qualities such as confidence, good communication skills, empathy, compassion and having the ability to learn, as well as having the capacity to reflect, creates an excellent foundation on which any nurse can build to become successful.

Becoming a CNS is no different. Good foundations are important. It is necessary for any CNS to have a good all-round experience of general nursing in either medicine or surgery, or possibly both, before deciding to specialize. In making that decision, that individual nurse needs to develop a heightened knowledge base in his or her chosen sphere of nursing, and continue learning to facilitate becoming an expert within that specialty. I would suggest that in order to be a successful clinical nurse specialist, you need:

- the ability to learn
- the ability to reflect on yourself, evaluating what you are good at and what things could be improved on
- to be a good communicator, skilful, empathetic, knowledgeable
- to be honest and truthful with yourself and others
- diplomacy
- strategic vision and the determination to succeed
- to be organized and able to prioritize
- confidence in your own judgment and decision-making.

The role

According to Hamric and Spross (1989), there are specific competencies and subroles for any CNS. These include:

- clinical practice
- leadership/management

Career destinations – clinical nurse specialist

- consultant
- collaborator
- educator
- researcher.

Having such varied aspects to the role encourages daily diversity. Having a strong clinical component to the role is a high priority for any nurse. Many CNSs care for the whole age spectrum, so as a CNS you might be caring for:

- a premature baby in the special care baby unit, providing the support and information required by his anxious parents
- a moody, uncommunicative adolescent who won't listen to any healthcare professional
- a middle-aged woman who has just been informed that she has a cancer and may well need body-altering surgery to try to cure her disease
- an older person who has been told she is dying.

Caring for such a wide range of age groups and helping patients understand numerous wide-ranging disease processes requires a myriad of skills, which are often not learnt, but acquired by experience and simply by being there.

Building relationships with patients

In many specialties the CNS is the key individual who meets the patient at the beginning of their care pathway and supports them and their relatives throughout the whole journey. This relationship often begins to develop in the outpatient clinic. In most specialties, the CNS will generally see patients as both inpatients and outpatients. Patients will regularly consult with the CNS, making him or her the initial point of contact for information, whether it's about their clinical condition or arrangements for appointments. In some specialties, this bond expands further, as some CNSs have a pivotal role linking acute hospital care with primary care. Depending on the specialty, some CNSs encourage and support the development of user/support

patients will **regularly consult** with the **clinical** **nurse specialist**

groups as a means of helping patients cope with a diagnosis or a change in body image or lifestyle.

Nurse-led clinics

Many CNSs also run independent nurse-led clinics. In such clinics, existing patients are reviewed solely by the CNS and treatment decisions are made. CNSs are autonomous practitioners; they are confident and competent to make independent decisions, particularly within their own specialist sphere of practice. In some situations, a discussion with a medical colleague may be necessary, but invariably this is not essential. In recent years, there has been much discussion about nurse prescribing, and it is encouraging that many nurses are now able to prescribe from a specific formulary. Many hospital-based CNSs use a patient group direction (PGD) as a guide for treating specific patients with a specific problem. For example, a CNS in stoma care may use a PGD for hydrocortisone to treat an obvious product allergy in his or her nurse-led clinic and will review the effects a week later.

Providing education

Education is an important part of the CNS role. It is vital to share knowledge and encourage good, effective and evidence-based practice. The CNS is involved in numerous teaching scenarios. These include informal teaching to other healthcare professionals in clinical situations on the ward and in more formal settings, within universities and on specialist courses, as well as educating patients, carers and their families.

education is an important part of the role

Research

Many CNSs are involved with both primary research and research carried out collaboratively with commercial companies. Such involvement helps to ensure that products or drugs are effective, efficient, and fulfil the majority of patients' needs.

There are some obvious social benefits to being a CNS – there's no shift work and you work very few weekends. On a negative note, most CNSs work long hours as, unlike the situation with ward work, there is no one to 'hand over' to – all the necessary care and documentation needs to be completed by the CNS and it is often not feasible to leave tasks until the following day. Therefore, being organized and having the ability to prioritize is paramount for a CNS.

Obviously one disadvantage to advancing the role of a CNS is the added documentation and protocols that are needed. Writing such protocols can be immensely time-consuming. However, undoubtedly for any CNS, the reward is being given the opportunity to provide the best possible care to their patients – and that reward is beyond measure.

Voice of experience
The clinical nurse specialist

- Be organized and ensure you are able to prioritize your workload efficiently and effectively for your patients and yourself!
- Listen carefully, with your ears (and your eyes!), to what a patient is saying
- Ongoing education is vital for advancing your own knowledge base/practice, so adopt the concept of lifelong learning
- Be confident in your own judgments and decision-making, but if you don't know, don't be afraid to admit it and ask for help
- Plan, write and evaluate all the advancements to your role, highlighting dates that you achieved a competence – it's essential for specialist nurses to initiate advancing roles and have a strategic vision for role/service development
- Keep rigorously to protocols and guidelines to ensure that patients get safe, evidence-based and effective care

Further reading

Hamric A, Spross J. *The Clinical Nurse Specialist in Theory and Practice*, 2nd edn. Philadelphia: WB Saunders, 1989.

The United Kingdom Central Council for Nursing, Midwifery and Health Visiting. *The Scope of Professional Practice.* London: UKCC, 1992 (available from www.xxxxx.dircon.co.uk/scope.htm). Note that this has now been replaced by: Nursing and Midwifery Council. *The NMC Code of Professional Conduct: Standards for Conduct, Performance and Ethics.* NMC: London, 2004 (available from www.nmc-uk.org).

modern matron

Amy Gass, Former Matron,
General and Vascular Surgery, and currently
Head of Nursing for Surgery,
St George's Healthcare NHS Trust, London

Many nurses simply enjoy working on a ward, caring for patients; others enjoy the challenge of managing a team of staff or a department as a sister or charge nurse. If the latter is you, you may plan to move up to the role of matron, which was brought back by the government in 2000 as part of the NHS Plan (Department of Health 2000, 2002).

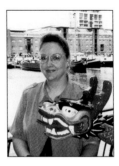

A matron usually manages several ward or outpatient areas, though he or she may also manage one very large area such as accident and emergency. The matron is professionally accountable to the head of nursing in his or her directorate or to the director of nursing on the trust board, depending on the organization's structure. A matron's line manager may be a senior nurse or a service manager. Typically, ward/outpatient sisters and charge nurses, as well as some clinical nurse specialists, report to a matron. In some areas, administrative staff may also report to a matron.

> a matron usually manages several ward or outpatient areas

I have worked in a variety of hospitals, both in London and Australia, and I followed a traditional pathway of staff nurse to sister. In August 2001, I was appointed as the first matron at St George's Healthcare NHS Trust, a London teaching hospital. I was very excited to be one of the first matrons and to have an opportunity to drive up standards of care in the area I was managing and to be seen to be making a difference to patients' experiences. I had the opportunity to make changes that would influence peoples' perceptions of the role in a positive way.

Becoming a matron

Being a matron is all about being a strong clinical leader with clear authority. Therefore, it is important that you have well-developed clinical leadership skills, excellent communication and interpersonal skills, and the ability to influence and implement change. You should be self-motivated, confident in your abilities and able to work independently and as part of a team.

being a matron is all about being a **strong clinical leader** with **clear authority**

If you have had experience of both managing a team of staff at ward or department level, and of working in a multidisciplinary team, and you feel ready for a different challenge, you could consider becoming a matron. Continuously improving quality should be top of your agenda. But it will also be important to take a corporate view at times, rather than just working locally, so you should be prepared to work on trust-wide projects, developing policies and procedures that affect a wide area.

Key responsibilities

The key responsibilities of matrons were outlined by the government from the outset (see Table 1). The day-to-day job involves all of these key responsibilities and I'll discuss how, as a matron, you can successfully meet these.

Leading by example

As a matron, you are a visible clinical leader – you might find yourself in a clinical area discussing aspects of nursing care, teaching staff, investigating complaints or conducting audits of the environment. Personally, I have never expected staff do anything that I would not do

Table 1

- Leading by example
- Making sure patients get quality care
- Ensuring staffing is appropriate to patient needs
- Empowering nurses to take on a wider range of clinical tasks
- Improving hospital cleanliness
- Ensuring patients' nutritional needs are met
- Improving wards for patients
- Making sure patients are treated with respect
- Preventing hospital-acquired infection
- Resolving problems for patients and their relatives by building closer relationships

myself, so when I worked as a matron I cleaned toilets and made cups of tea for patients when the circumstances required.

Making sure patients get quality care

One of the ways to make sure patients get quality care is to try to minimize clinical risk. The clinical risk agenda grows ever greater, with the National Patient Safety Agency (NPSA) as well as the Medicines and Healthcare products Regulatory Agency (MHRA) producing alerts and information about reducing clinical risk. As a learning organization, the NHS is getting much better at understanding why mistakes are

> the clinical risk agenda grows ever greater

happening. As a matron, you contribute to that process by analysing adverse incident forms to find the root cause of why an incident occurred, and then taking the appropriate steps to try to prevent similar incidents. This information is fed into the trust's database which, in turn, informs the NPSA. For example, an incident form about a drug error by a nurse had as its root cause an an unusual drug regimen prescribed by a doctor. It is important that staff feel able to tell you exactly what happened and that they can do this in a blame-free way. Obviously, to get the most accurate information, it is helpful to investigate the incident as soon as possible after it happened and for staff to keep good records.

Health and safety is also important. You are responsible for making sure that health and safety legislation and policies are followed in the areas you manage. Audits and risk assessments are carried out in conjunction with the ward/department sisters and charge nurses: for example, you look at the use of computer workstations, hazardous substances and sharps, and identify dangerous work practices. As part of this, you have to identify the action that should be taken to correct any deficits. This might include referrals to estate departments or medical physics departments for the repairs to the fabric of the building or to medical equipment, respectively.

investigate the incident as soon as possible after it happened

Surveying patient satisfaction is another method of measuring quality. Sometimes this is done by asking patients to complete diaries, but more commonly they are asked to complete questionnaires. Patient satisfaction scores are going to be increasingly important as patients choose more of their healthcare options. As a matron, you may have to analyse the data from such questionnaires. In one such survey, I found that patients wanted more information about their diagnoses and operations. With this information, we were able to develop patient information leaflets for a range of conditions.

A friend and former line manager, Amanda Payne, once said "Good communication shows you care, good documentation proves it." You need to be able to demonstrate that care given to a patient is based on evidence-based practice. As a matron, you have a role in developing and updating existing ward care plans to ensure that they are evidence-based. And you'll also be involved in developing trust policies and procedures that are relevant to your sphere of practice. This requires written communication skills that can be developed as a staff nurse (though nurses at all levels can contribute to the development of policies and procedures). Typically, for this part of the role, you would have to conduct literature searches, apply relevant findings, and then document the evidence-based care in the trust's preferred documentation styles. You would also present any policies/procedures for ratification within the department or organization.

Resolving problems for patients and their relatives

Resolving problems for patients and their relatives is essential for preventing complaints, formal or informal. While it is preferable to be proactive in preventing complaints by delivering high-quality care and communicating in a caring, honest and timely manner with patients and relatives, it is also necessary to investigate and respond to any formal or informal complaints that come your way. Formal complaints come through the trust's quality improvement department, but you may also be called to the ward or outpatients or be contacted by the Patient Advice and Liaison Service (PALS). Investigating the complaints may involve listening to patients and/or relatives, and taking action where necessary to provide information or to change something. It also involves apologizing for how people feel and saying sorry when the organization has got it wrong.

Making sure patients are treated with respect

All patients deserve to be treated with respect – they should be addressed in the way they choose and their privacy and dignity should be maintained. As a matron you will be involved in auditing against the *Essence of Care* privacy and dignity benchmarks (Modernisation Agency 2003) and in promoting best practice. Matrons around the country have already been involved in initiatives to improve curtains (e.g. by using tapes or pegs to keep them shut when around bed spaces) and in redesigning theatre gowns.

all patients deserve to be treated with respect

Meeting nutritional needs

Nutrition is highly valued on today's wards although many patients are still leaving hospital malnourished. As a matron, you can contribute at trust level by being on the nutritional strategy groups and implementing the good practice outlined in the *Essence of Care* standards, such as protecting meal times and making sure patients get assistance with feeding if they need it.

Ensuring staffing is appropriate to patient need

To maintain a safe level of care, it is important that wards and departments have sufficient staff with the correct skills. As the matron, you are involved in recruiting and selecting staff, interviewing staff after sickness absences, and appraising staff performance. Make sure you discuss staffing levels with sisters/charge nurses so you can ensure they have sufficient staff. If patients' needs have changed or you expect them to change (e.g. you anticipate more complex surgery being done), then you should negotiate having extra staff with managers, particularly during the budget-setting process, which usually occurs in the autumn. Also, during the business planning cycle, you may be required to calculate the nurses needed to set up a new service or change an existing one – you would work closely with business or service managers on this.

become **involved** in **internal staff development programmes**

In order to make sure staff have the right skills, encourage them to develop themselves. Support them to pursue study that's appropriate to their needs and also to the needs of the ward or outpatient department. Become involved in internal staff development programmes and work to develop links with the local university and training and development departments so that the training and development opportunities meet the needs of your staff.

Empowering nurses

Clinical nurse specialists traditionally take on a wider range of tasks, some developing specialist skills in diagnosing conditions and prescribing care. You need to make sure that they are developing their practice but you also need to look to see where a specialist role might enhance the existing services. This is being influenced currently by the changes in junior doctor training and hours, with the development of more practitioner roles. Spotting gaps and opportunities is important for business planning.

Improving cleanliness

One of my biggest achievements was, with a few other matrons, setting up MEATe, the Matrons Environmental Action Team, within the trust in which I worked. This brought together matrons with facilities and estates staff to discuss and resolve issues of cleanliness and the environment. I was also involved in the tendering process for a new cleaning contract as a result of this and met with potential companies to articulate my expectations of a future provider of

you can, and should, be getting things done

cleaning services. As a matron, you can, and should, be getting things done, turning around poor practice if it exists. And hospital cleanliness, which seems to be forever in the headlines, is an area on which you'll have to focus.

At ward level, you'll be involved in auditing the cleanliness of the environment and in dealing with the domestic staff to sort out problems as they arise. It is frustrating when cleaning improves in the short term only to deteriorate again. You need to keep a close eye on what's happening and you need to report issues to higher managers when the problems are not resolved locally. But it helps if the domestic staff are made to feel part of the ward team and are invited to ward meetings (so they have an opportunity to voice problems too) and are present at cleaning audits so that they can see how their work impacts on maintaining a clean and safe environment for patients.

Improving wards for patients

There is a lot of research now available about the importance of the healing environment. Changing lighting, introducing plants or changing views can go part of the way to creating that healing environment. The government has a ward-improvement fund which allows ward sisters/charge nurses a sum of money to spend as they see fit, and even small changes can have a big impact. One day, when I was touring a ward, a patient commented that, as he'd spent a lot of time lying on his back in bed and looking upwards, he'd noticed an accumulation of dead flies in the fluorescent lighting. Once estates staff had cleaned the ward lights, everyone commented on how much brighter the ward appeared. Similarly, adding a few artificial plants into a windowless space in clinic and decluttering noticeboards and walls can improve outpatient environments significantly. And improving the environment doesn't just benefit patients. Staff morale can increase greatly as well.

improving the environment doesn't just benefit patients

Preventing hospital-acquired infection

The government has placed great emphasis on reducing hospital-acquired infection. In 2004, *A Matron's Charter* (Department of Health 2004) was issued laying out a number of key objectives. In clinical practice, the matron not only has to act as a role model to staff, but also needs to observe the practice of staff and give feedback. This might be done by doing a simple 30-minute observation of care which looks at ward events during a set time period and gives immediate feedback to staff or by working a clinical shift on a ward. The matron also has to look at how systems are working in a particular department (e.g. storage of sterile/non-sterile goods, and the location of handwashing facilities) and monitor levels of cleanliness. Where audits have been carried out, it is also important that recommendations are acted on – you have to liaise closely with the infection control team to address any concerns.

- Read about the medical and nursing care of the specialty you are working in and make the most of any orientation period to ask questions of the people that you meet – at this stage, you don't know what you don't know, so asking questions is a way of establishing what you need to know
- Work safely, following policies and procedures, and don't be afraid to ask if you don't know how to do something. If you cut corners, before long you'll make a mistake
- Communicate, communicate and communicate – put yourself in the patients' and visitors' shoes to see it from their point of view
- Maintain good records, both patient records and records of your own personal development
- Look after yourself – take regular breaks during your shift because your brain needs energy and water to keep it performing well. Spread your annual leave throughout the year to prevent tiredness and burnout too
- Make time to learn something new – whether from a journal, book, the Internet or from study days, and then reflect on how it applies to your practice

Further reading

Department of Health. *NHS Plan: A Plan For Investment, A Plan For Reform.* London: TSO, 2000 (available from www.dh.gov.uk).

Department of Health. *Modern Matrons in the NHS: A Progress Report.* London: TSO, 2002 (available from www.dh.gov.uk).

Department of Health. *A Matron's Charter: An Action Plan for Cleaner Hospitals.* London: TSO, 2004 (available from www.nhsestates.gov.uk).

Modernisation Agency. *Essence of Care – Patient-focused Benchmarking for Health Care Practitioners.* London: TSO, 2003 (available from www.modern.nhs.uk).

nursing in the community
- the practice nurse

Anne Hitchen, Practice Nurse,
Broken Cross Surgery,
Macclesfield

Nurses working in general practice can be traced back as far as 1913 – Hannah Mary Robson was working in Northumberland for a Dr Grant. Hannah Mary dispensed medicine, changed dressings and took out-of-hours calls, deciding which could be dealt with by herself or the doctor – an enlightened woman of the time.

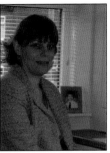

Up until the 1970s, a few GPs employed nurses. They were based in the treatment room and dealt with dressings and syringed blocked ears. In the early 80s, a government report, *Neighbourhood Nursing – a Focus for Care*, suggested that nurses were not needed in general practice, and that the work could be carried out by "community practitioners" attached to the surgery. This caused a national outcry from practice nurses, who wanted to continue to be employed in general practice. They were spurred into action, and by the end of the 80s, the role of nursing in general practice was expanding to include phlebotomy, cervical cytology, electrocardiography and immunizations. Nurses were pushing the boundaries with endless enthusiasm and taking on chronic diseases such as asthma and diabetes. There were no formal educational courses, and many nurses either self-funded or appealed to pharmaceutical

> nurses working in general practice can be traced back as far as 1913

company reps for funding to attend courses in the areas in which they were interested.

In 1990, the government introduced the new GP contract. GPs were to be paid for services such as new patient checks, health assessments for over-75s, health promotion and minor surgery. There were also targets to meet for childhood immunization and cervical cytology. GPs quickly realized that to have a nurse to carry out this work for them was to their advantage, and the numbers of practice nurses swelled. The nurses themselves were realizing that, in order to take on the extended role required of them, they needed education to underpin their experience.

A 28-day basic training course was developed by the English National Board, with an attendance certificate supplied at the end. But this was not really enough to satisfy practice nurses, plus the tutors had no real idea of the practice nurse role, being from district nursing or health visiting backgrounds.

The Royal College of Nursing (RCN) lobbied the United Kingdom Central Council for Nursing, Midwifery and Health Visiting (the UKCC) and worked tirelessly to ensure that practice nurses gained training opportunities equal to those available for their district nurse and health visitor colleagues. Today, we have nurses accessing the degree programme leading to a specialist practitioner qualification in general practice nursing. This gives practice nurses a recordable qualification and it means they can apply theory to practice on a higher academic level and use evidence-based practice in their day-to-day work.

Moving into practice nursing

The majority of practice nurses are employed by GPs rather than primary care trusts (PCTs). It's this that makes the role so different – there is no hierarchical structure to follow. Many practice nurses value the autonomy of the role, and the freedom to be innovative for the benefit of the patients.

Practice nursing tends to attract nurses with families as the hours are easier to fit around children, with no shifts or weekend working. Having said that, the role is attracting younger nurses, and this is possibly because pre-registration student nurses spend time in the community observing all areas of primary healthcare.

There are many ways to become a practice nurse: you can of course apply for an advertised post. But most jobs require the applicant to have relevant experience as a practice nurse first. If you're starting out, it's probably advisable to apply for a lower-grade post in a team so that you can gain clinical experience over time with good support from the rest of the nursing team (you need experience in many areas – cervical cytology, travel medicine, immunization and vaccination, chronic disease management, and family planning). Or you can apply to undertake the degree programme to obtain the specialist practitioner qualification, which would give you the theory but possibly not a lot of practice – having this might mean you could go into a higher grade, but once there, you might not necessarily have the experience to back it up. I would estimate that the majority of nurses working in general practice got the experience first and then applied for a higher-grade post.

> **most jobs** require the **applicant** to have **relevant experience** as a **practice nurse**

Contracts, accountability and pension

If you're entering general practice, make sure you have a contract with terms and conditions clearly stated (the RCN has several helpful publications on its website). A job description is essential, and you must ensure you have the professional competency to carry out what is required. As nurses, we are accountable for our actions as laid down by our professional body, the Nursing and Midwifery Council. If coming from NHS employment, pension rights can be transferred into general practice and carried on.

Professional development

Practice nurses are able to attend the nurse prescribing course, enabling them to prescribe from the *Nurse Prescriber's Extended Formulary*. This means they can prescribe treatments for minor illnesses and treat conditions relevant to their clinical practice, such as diabetes or asthma, as a supplementary prescriber, using clinical management plans agreed with the patient and doctor. The training helps nurses to:

- understand influences in prescribing practice
- understand the legislation relevant to nurse prescribing
- apply knowledge of drugs and their actions
- prescribe safely and appropriately
- undertake assessment and consultation with patients.

There are also nurse practitioners working in general practice who have studied to masters level and who see and treat patients for minor illness or chronic disease.

Life in the community

The first thing to say is that no two days are ever the same when you work in the community! The best advice I can give to a nurse contemplating moving into practice nursing is to be prepared for the unexpected, always have a smile on your face, and if you cannot sort out the patient's presenting problem then find someone who can. Plenty of common sense is an essential requirement as is, most important of all, a good sense of humour! Practice nurses can either work alone or as part of a team, depending on the size of the practice. To be a practice nurse, you need to enjoy meeting and talking to people from all walks of life.

A typical surgery for a practice nurse might involve consultations for:

- hypertension management – this would mean checking the patient's blood pressure and medication compliance, and giving dietary and smoking advice
- dressings (e.g. changing a dressing for a leg ulcer)
- a cervical smear
- contraceptives (including requests for emergency contraception)
- statin therapy
- rheumatology monitoring
- travel advice.

There may also be lunchtime triage of calls for urgent appointments/advice (not all surgeries do this) and liaison with the health visitor or district nurse.

Expect the unexpected

When you work in the community, you should always expect the unexpected. Don't put your patients off by saying you haven't got time to sort out other problems – they might not come back to see you again. For example, if a patient attending for contraception advice mentions that she wants to give up smoking, you have to make time to chat about it and refer her to the appropriate professional, rather than saying you haven't got time to talk about it.

Our role is holistic in the truest sense and you look at the patient as a whole and not just as a 'problem' to be dealt with. Working in the hospital setting means you see a patient, nurse him for a short while until he is better, discharge him and probably never see him again, whereas in general practice you might see the patient, his wife, his children, the whole family! This is true primary healthcare and it gives so much opportunity to offer health promotion and advice in a friendly

you look at the patient as a whole

and non-judgmental way. It's satisfying when you overhear a patient saying that they enjoy their visits to the surgery; you know then that you're doing a good job.

Information and support

Some days you feel like a trouble-shooter (I have been described as this), with people asking you for all sorts of advice and help. You need to have a broad knowledge base. There are many websites available to support you, so an understanding of the Internet helps. Nurses can access travel health sites, the Department of Health website, the RCN site, and sites specific for practice nurses – the list is endless (Table 1). To be computer literate is a bonus as most, if not all, practices now use computers routinely. Although they all use different operating systems, to be able to know your way around a computer helps enormously.

There are also many community-focused journals and magazines with up-to-date articles and information that can be really helpful and relevant to practice nurses.

Table 1

Some helpful starting points for information

- **www.practicenursing.co.uk**
- **www.practicenurse.org.uk**
- **www.rcn.org.uk** for information from the Royal College of Nursing
- **www.dh.gov.uk** for information from the Department of Health
- **www.prodigy.nhs.uk**
- **www.earcarecentre.com** for information on all aspects of ear care
- **www.nathnac.org** for travel health and advice

Working with the health visitor and district nurse

The roles of practice nurse, health visitor and district nurse differ vastly and can also vary from practice to practice. Health visitors and district nurses are employed by the PCT. At my own practice, the health visitors see the under-5s for developmental checks, immunizations and advice. They are also involved in coronary rehabilitation (seeing patients who have had a heart attack, who get advice and support for a period of time once discharged from hospital). Our district nurses visit and care for patients at home. It's essential to have a good working relationship with your colleagues so you can liaise about patients over whom you, or they, have concerns.

If problems arise at work

Speak out if you are unhappy about any aspect of the role. And if you are asked to do something for which you have not been trained, don't do it. You might want to refer back to the terms and conditions of your employment or to the professional code of conduct. It's also a good idea to talk to other practice nurses and find out what they do or contact your local RCN representative for further advice. Finally, remember that GPs want to keep their practice nurses happy. Your decisions should be respected, and training needs and opportunities should be discussed with you at your annual appraisal.

Future directions and opportunities

Practice nursing has moved so fast over the last decade that it's hard to keep pace. The role is expanding all the time and we now have nurse prescribers, nurse practitioners taking on minor illness and chronic disease management, community matrons, first-contact care ... the list is endless.

The new general medical services contract for doctors in general practice means that GPs are becoming more proactive than reactive and

Voice of experience

The practice nurse

- Smile
- Study
- Read practice nursing magazines and journals to keep up to date
- Attend relevant courses whenever possible – your practice should fund you if it is relevant/essential for you to perform your role; the local PCT will also have training opportunities, and if they have a practice nurse facilitator in post she will have up-to-date information on courses and funding
- Speak out if you are unhappy about any aspect of the role
- Get to know your patients well (though this can be a nuisance when they see you in the supermarket and shout "There's our nurse, doesn't she look different with her clothes on!" – you can get some very strange looks!)
- Join the local practice nurse forum/group – these are usually very active and can act as a voice within the local PCT; we work within multidisciplinary teams but value our autonomy highly in the general practice setting (it is important to maintain the links with the PCTs but also to keep our independence)
- Check out the websites available and join the RCN Practice Nurse Association, which holds annual conferences that are devoted entirely to practice nursing – this keeps you abreast with what's going on politically

the emphasis has shifted to prevention and management of chronic disease, with many practice nurses taking the lead in these areas. We're starting to see partnerships with GPs, nurse-led surgeries, and nurses employing doctors. Watch out, practice nurses are taking over!

mental health nursing

Ben Thomas, Director of Nursing and Organisational
Development, Somerset Partnership NHS and
Social Care Trust, and Senior Lecturer,
University of Plymouth. On secondment as
Chief Nurse to St Vincent's Mental Health Services,
Melbourne, Australia (2003–05)

At any one time in the UK, one adult in six suffers from one or other form of mental illness. Mental health nurses provide the majority of professional care required by people with a mental illness, in a variety of settings. People often think of mental health nursing as a single specialty. However, there are many specialist areas within mental health nursing and as a mental health nurse, you could be looking after people of all ages and backgrounds. Many of the specialist areas have

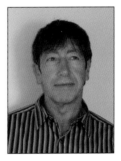

their own additional training courses to prepare nurses to work with particular client groups. These specialist areas include:

- forensic care (working with people who have a mental illness, have committed a crime and are remanded in custody, for example in a prison or forensic psychiatric hospital)
- liaison psychiatry (working with people who have a physical illness and mental health problems)
- children and adolescents
- people who use drugs and alcohol
- older people.

Student nurses are often fortunate enough to be able to

> there are **many specialist areas** within **mental health nursing**

undertake a placement in many of these specialist areas so they can experience working first hand with particular client groups.

The role

As a first-level mental health nurse you can pursue a career rich in diversity and opportunity within a range of employment settings. In the inpatient setting, mental health nurses provide direct care and also coordinate the delivery of care by others. Similarly, in the community the mental health nurse is often the coordinator of care and is known as the case manager. This involves collaborating and negotiating with other professionals. The nurse works as part of a multidisciplinary team while being individually accountable and responsible for the care he or she delivers. Mental health nurses develop therapeutic relationships with service users and their carers through open, honest and purposeful communication. This is the cornerstone of mental health nursing, where the service user is seen as central to service provision and where nursing care is tailored to individual needs, including a person's culture, ethnicity, gender, sexuality and religion.

the **service user** is seen as **central** to **service provision**

Nurses carry out comprehensive assessments of service users' needs. Mental health nurses take a holistic approach to patient care and whereas the nursing assessment may contribute to diagnosing the patient, and often involves carrying out a 'mental state examination', the nurse is particularly concerned with the patient's individual experience of illness, expression of symptoms and their response to treatment. Nurses develop effective interventions and implement a plan of nursing care. The nursing interventions are aimed at meeting psychosocial and physical health needs as well as mental health promotion. Nursing interventions include highly developed communication skills, a range of psychosocial approaches, such as cognitive behavioural therapy and family therapy, the administration of medication and the monitoring of side effects.

Mental health nurses also have legal functions. Under the Mental Health Act 1983, a first-level mental health nurse may detain a patient in a ward or department of a hospital in specific circumstances. The nurse's holding power is intended to prevent harm and to detain a patient long enough for a risk assessment to be carried out by a medical practitioner.

The draft Mental Health Bill which, as I write, is undergoing pre-legislative scrutiny by a parliamentary committee with a report expected in Spring 2005, is designed to be compatible with the European Convention on Human Rights by giving patients more choice and autonomy. However, there are a number of contentious changes suggested in the new Bill, not least that mental health nurses may be eligible to undertake new roles such as Approved Mental Health Professional (AMHP), the clinical member of the tribunal or the clinical supervisor (i.e. the professional in charge of the care of a person detained under the Bill).

Becoming a mental health nurse

Pre-registration preparation

Traditionally in the UK, mental health nursing training programmes were direct entry and of 3-year duration. However, with the introduction of Project 2000 and the transfer of nurse training into higher education, the direct entry courses were phased out and replaced with a split programme comprising an 18-month common foundation programme followed by a further 18-month mental health branch component. The greater emphasis on general nursing at the expense of mental health nursing resulted in questions being raised as to whether mental health nurses trained under this system were adequately skilled and knowledgeable to undertake the role. Mental health nurse training underwent further reforms and by 1999 the current system was introduced, with a 1-year common foundation programme and a 2-year mental health branch component.

Current requirements

To become a mental health nurse, you need to complete the common foundation programme (CFP), which provides an introduction to the principles of nursing practice and normally takes 12 months to complete. During this time there are exams and practical assessments. The mental health branch training, which takes about 2 years, builds on the knowledge and skills acquired during the CFP. There is normally a choice of completing the training at degree or diploma level. The diploma of higher education nursing (Dip HE Nursing) is usually a 3-year course divided into theory and supervised clinical practice. The degree in nursing may take 3 or 4 years according to the number of study weeks. First-level nurses in the UK must be registered with the Nursing and Midwifery Council. Most nursing educational pathways provide a structure that allows nurses to choose from a variety of academic awards, from diplomas to PhDs.

After qualifying

Traditionally, most mental health nurses work on acute psychiatric wards after they have qualified. Recently, this way of gaining experience has been questioned. First, because of the shift from hospital to the community as the major setting for mental healthcare, and second because of the increasingly specialist and expert nature of nursing on acute wards. Whereas most mental health problems are treated at primary care level, services do not seem able, as yet, to take on the responsibility for training mental health nurses. In the meantime, the level of skills required to work on acute psychiatric wards has been formally recognized in recent years and a number of specialist courses are being developed to help nurses work more therapeutically with people admitted to hospital.

There are, of course, a number of arguments to support most postgraduates continuing to gain a good deal of their work experience on acute psychiatric wards. First, in a ward situation newly qualified nurses have a built-in support system in terms of their colleagues in the immediate environment. Therefore, nurses are more likely to be able to check things out with other members of staff, have supervision and mentorship, and find a 'safety net' when situations are difficult. Second, the mix of patients on an acute ward means that nurses gain practical experience caring for a variety of people with difficult-to-manage behaviour and they are exposed to a number of complex situations. Third, there is an opportunity to work at an organizational level, which can provide role modelling, training opportunities, motivation for continuing development and other benefits not always acknowledged or appreciated when working in a more independent, autonomous way.

in a **ward situation** newly qualified nurses have a **built-in support system**

The 'specialist–generic debate' continues to generate interest among the profession. Recent government initiatives aimed at bringing closer the working relationships between mental health professionals and social services are seen by some as an opportunity for mental health nurses to distance themselves from general nursing and develop the role of a specialized 'mental health worker'.

Obviously there are some benefits for service users in terms of the specialist skills and knowledge of the 'mental health worker'. There is also a common knowledge base and competencies that underpin all those professional groups who care for people with a mental illness. Recently these competencies have been clearly articulated and some of them are shared with other professional groups. However, many remain specific to mental health nursing, not least the ability to promote and maintain service users' physical well-being. In addition to knowledge and competencies, it is important for mental health nurses to be aware of their own values and to have positive attitudes towards people with a mental illness so that they are treated with respect and dignity at all times. As our knowledge base increases in mental health and we become more skilled in different therapeutic interventions, so the need for more in-depth understanding and additional training increases. For example, after qualifying I undertook a number of training courses in facilitating groups and group analysis, which enabled me to facilitate groups both on inpatient units and in the community. The development of the nurse consultant role often calls for clinical expertise and specialist skills in particular areas such as cognitive behaviour and psychosocial interventions therapy.

> it is **important** to be aware of your own values

A continuum of care

Meeting the needs of people with mental health problems requires the input of several professionals and a range of services, and these are normally arranged along a continuum of care. This is often referred to as a spectrum of care and treatment (Figure 1). In recent years the prevention of mental illness, despite its complexities, has been added to this spectrum. It now includes preventive measures targeted at whole population groups, individuals or a subgroup of the population whose risk of developing a disorder is higher than average and/or high-risk individuals indicating a predisposition to a mental disorder. This is an exciting and developing field, but so far mental health nurses have been slow to realize the enormous contribution they could make in this area.

Some of the issues on the horizon for mental health nurses are summarized in Table 1.

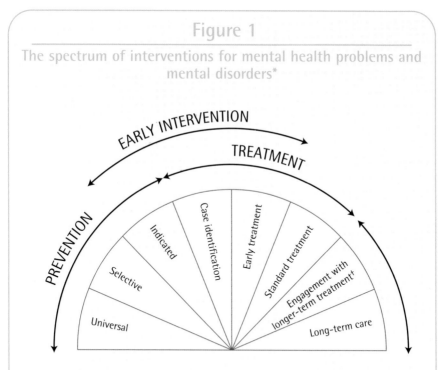

Figure 1

The spectrum of interventions for mental health problems and mental disorders*

EARLY INTERVENTION

TREATMENT

PREVENTION

Indicated

Case identification

Early treatment

Standard treatment

Engagement with longer-term treatment†

Selective

Universal

Long-term care

†Including relapse prevention

*Reprinted with permission from National Academy of Sciences. *Reducing Risks for Mental Disorders: Frontiers for Preventive Intervention Research.* Washington DC: National Academies Press, 1994

Table 1

On the horizon for mental health nurses

- A huge part to play in shaping and delivering modern mental health services
- An extended role – taking on work traditionally seen as the province of other disciplines, such as the supplementary prescribing of medication
- A rediscovery of some previous roles not recently in vogue, such as facilitating groups, particularly in inpatient settings
- Recognition of the implications of an ageing population for mental health services (for example, at the moment we know very little about the needs of people diagnosed with schizophrenia as they grow older)
- A greater role in mental health promotion – the prominent position nurses have to play in targeting individuals, communities and populations will be identified as knowledge and strategies around prevention become commonplace
- An increase in confidence and a growing political awareness at national and international levels to ensure that the front-line role of mental health nurses is strengthened

The Australian experience

While writing this piece, I have been on a 2-year secondment in Australia, as Chief Nurse to St Vincent's Mental Health Services, Melbourne. Although I've had to learn about a different health system and a different educational system, I've been grappling with many of the same nursing problems that are common in the UK. Unlike the UK system where mental health trusts are separate entities to acute trusts, in Victoria mental health services have been 'mainstreamed' into general health settings and co-located with acute hospitals. The benefits of such a system include the reduction of stigma sometimes associated with the use of mental health services and the provision of a single point of entry through psychiatric triage, which is normally situated in general hospital emergency departments. The main difference in training to be a psychiatric nurse is that, unlike the UK system, in Victoria registered nurses have to complete a bachelor of nursing degree. Those wishing to work as mental health nurses are then encouraged and supported to undertake a graduate year programme or a postgraduate course in mental health nursing. This secondment is the kind of opportunity that can present itself. Mental health nursing can provide individuals with a challenging, satisfying and rewarding career. With a little creativity and imagination, you can shape your own career, whatever your idea of success.

Voice of experience
The mental health nurse

- Always put the service user at the centre of everything you do – the relationship between you and the service user is the medium for all therapeutic interventions
- Be clear about your values and let them underpin your day-to-day work – your own values are as important as anything else you bring to mental healthcare
- Pursue postgraduate education and training, and be prepared to learn and take advantage of every opportunity – let lifelong learning be a reality
- Ensure you have clinical supervision and learn from self-reflection
- Find a good role model, particularly in the clinical area; observe not only the way they interact with service users but how they handle their own emotions

Further reading

Department of Health. *The Mental Health Policy Guide.* London: TSO, 2001.

Department of Health. *Mental Health Policy Implementation Guide: Adult Acute Inpatient Care Provision.* London: TSO, 2002.

nursing in the
independent sector

Linda Nazarko, Nurse Consultant – Older People,
Richmond and Twickenham Primary Care Trust, and
Visiting Senior Lecturer, King's College and London
South Bank Universities

The independent sector consists of private hospitals, nursing and residential homes (now known as care homes), new private walk-in centres and diagnostic treatment centres carrying out work under contract to the NHS. The sector has grown in the last 25 years – once there were only a few small private hospitals and small stand-alone nursing and residential homes. Most of the growth has been within care homes providing care and support to older people. These are mostly run as profit-making businesses; charities, local authorities and the NHS run the remainder. There are now 486 000 care-home beds and the care-home sector has twice as many beds as the NHS. Around a quarter of registered nurses work in the independent sector.

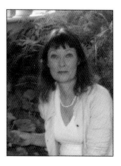

around a quarter of registered nurses work in the independent sector

Working in a care home

Most people living in care homes are older people, though some care homes care for younger people with specific needs such as learning disabilities or rehabilitation following brain injury. In the past, there were few checks on whether an older person required long-term care or what type of care was required. This changed with the introduction of the NHS and Community Care Act in 1993. Although people who are funding their own care can choose to enter a home if they wish, people who require state funding must now have their needs assessed. This assessment aims to determine the level of care required and where it can best be delivered. Government policy aims to enable older people to remain at home with appropriate support for as long as possible, and this has affected the level of care older people in care homes require.

Older people who require help with personal care are cared for in residential care homes. Care assistants staff these homes and there is no requirement for the home to employ registered nurses. If the person requires some nursing care, such as a dressing for a leg ulcer, a district nurse will visit and provide that care in the same way as if the person was living at home.

If a person requires a high level of nursing care, then nursing-home care is required. Nursing homes are the only places outside of hospital where registered nurses are on duty 24 hours a day to provide nursing care. Nurses work with care assistants to meet the residents' needs for nursing and personal care – on average, a quarter of nursing staff are registered nurses and three-quarters are care assistants.

People living in care homes require higher levels of care than ever before. Around two-thirds of people living in care homes have dementia. Some older people have mild dementia and an estimated one-third of people with dementia in care homes remain undiagnosed. In nursing homes, many people are now admitted in the last months or weeks of life and there is an increased emphasis on palliative care.

Table 1 gives some examples of the roles that nurses have in nursing homes today.

The qualities needed

Nurses considering a career in the care sector need to have a genuine respect for older people or the group being cared for, the ability to listen to older people and their families and a real desire to make a difference and provide high-quality care. These qualities are key – everything else can be learnt.

Table 1
Nursing roles in nursing homes

- Assessing older people prior to admission
- Assessing nursing and care needs on admission and on an ongoing basis
- Planning and managing care
- Providing rehabilitation and treatment
- Working with doctors to manage chronic disease
- Caring for people with end-stage disease
- Providing effective palliative care
- Working with other professionals to deliver care
- Supporting older people and their families
- Ensuring the home complies with legal standards
- Educating nursing and care staff
- Managing staff
- Managing budgets

The opportunities

Working in a care home appeals to lots of different nurses for different reasons. Some of the opportunities that can make nursing in a care home attractive are outlined below.

- You can really get to know the people you care for, and you can offer care that is truly tailored to the needs of individuals.
- Senior staff, such as the sister, deputy matron and matron, are often able to continue providing 'hands-on' care.
- There are usually opportunities to change things at ground level to improve the lives of residents (for example, if you notice that residents do not like some of the dishes on the menu, you can ask the home's chef to make some changes).
- The nursing roles offer variety, with opportunities to manage not just the nursing service but all other aspects of the day-to-day running of a home.
- There are opportunities to teach students nurses and NVQ students.

There are other reasons that nurses can find a care home an attractive place to work, many to do with maintaining the ever-important 'work/life balance'. More than 90% of registered nurses working in care homes are women, with over 50% working part-time. Many homes are in residential areas and people with domestic commitments can often find a position near to home with minimal travelling time. It's possible to obtain part-time posts at senior level with many homes, and this appeals to nurses with young children and those who are winding down their careers.

it's possible to obtain part-time posts at senior level with many homes

Career development

There are opportunities for nurses at all levels within care homes. You can work as a staff nurse, sister, deputy matron or matron/manager. In most homes, you'll need experience of working with older people and evidence of continued professional development to obtain posts at sister level and above. In England and Wales, matron/managers are now required to have an NVQ 4 or equivalent recognized management qualification. The Registered Nursing Home Association has developed a project to enable experienced matrons to gain this qualification using APEL (accreditation of prior experiential learning – learning that took place when doing the job). In Northern Ireland, new standards are about to be published but are not thought to require a recognized management qualification.

In some large care homes and in care home groups there are opportunities to work as a clinical nurse specialist in a particular clinical area, such as wound care, or as a nurse teacher. Teaching opportunities range from NVQ teachers, who teach and assess care assistants, to practice development nurses. Practice development nurses organize study days and teaching sessions and work with nurses in clinical practice, helping them to gain new skills such as suprapubic catheterization.

Nurses who wish to develop their management skills will find excellent opportunities for advancement within care homes. Nurses who have 2 years' relevant experience can work as matron/managers. Some matron/managers are provided with company cars, laptops and private medical insurance in addition to their salaries. Care home groups employ regional managers who support a group of care homes within a certain geographical area. The organization of this varies from group to group – some regional managers support a small number of large care homes within a small area, others support large numbers of smaller care homes over a larger area. Regional managers normally receive a comprehensive package that includes a company car and private medical insurance. There are also opportunities to manage the entire nursing service in a group of care homes, though not all large groups have director of nursing posts.

Where to work

The care home sector is a varied one. Most homes (75%) are run as small businesses and they are all different, so it's hard to make any general recommendations. It all comes down to your own preferences. And in addition to the stand-alone homes, there are the larger groups, such as BUPA and Westminster Health Care, that have hundreds of homes and well-developed management structures. If you work in a home that belongs to a group, you may find it more difficult to innovate and develop practice because you are expected to follow group-wide policies and procedures. But having said this, some groups encourage innovation and support staff in developing practice (and, in contrast, some small homes can be surprisingly rigid).

Nursing home groups tend to have modern, purpose-built homes that have been specifically adapted. You may find that these offer higher standards of accommodation for residents and more pleasant working conditions, or you may prefer the more 'homely' environment offered by a smaller home.

Advantages and disadvantages

Care homes can usually offer registered nurses great flexibility, so you can work part-time or keep to specific shifts if you wish.

On the potential downside, most care homes are not part of the NHS and are not obliged to pay NHS rates of pay or to offer NHS-type conditions. Pay and conditions vary enormously at all levels within care homes – for example, some care homes appear to offer rates that are higher than the NHS, but they don't pay supplements for unsocial hours. Many homes restrict the amount of sick pay staff can receive. And few care homes offer pension provision.

Employers within care homes vary in their willingness and ability to support nurses in continuing their education. Some employers will pay course fees and allow staff time off to attend courses. Other employers contribute to fees and time, while some employers make no contribution whatsoever. It is sensible to check a prospective employer's policy before accepting a post.

pay and conditions vary enormously

Another potential problem is that although nurses working in care homes are highly skilled, many report that these skills are often unrecognized when they apply for posts outside the care home sector. There are reports of matron/managers being forced to accept junior posts when moving back to the NHS. This is changing and there is increasing recognition of the skills and value of nurses working in care homes.

Future directions

The care home sector is changing and diversifying. Although most care homes continue to offer long-term care, intermediate care is becoming increasingly important. Some homes are now being set up and run solely to provide intermediate care under NHS contracts. These homes offer short-term rehabilitation to enable older people to recover as fully as possible following illness and accident and to return home. Some homes are now offering some intermediate care on a contract basis with the NHS. Some homes are also providing respite care so that the family of a frail older person living at home can have a break.

- Work out your career and life priorities
- Try to get some experience of working in a care home to see if you'd enjoy it – perhaps organize a few bank shifts
- Be aware of the dangers of professional isolation; read nursing journals, attend study days and continue to do relevant courses
- Consider doing a degree in gerontology if you wish to specialize in clinical practice
- If you wish to become a manager, obtain management qualifications

director of nursing

Denise Llewellyn, Executive Director of Nursing,
Carmarthenshire NHS Trust

An executive director of nursing in an acute trust has the opportunity not only to act as a nurse leading the nursing profession within a hospital setting but also to perform an executive role as a corporate member of the trust board. Being able to contribute strategically to both the professional and the strategic direction of the organization allows the postholder to influence patient care in a number of ways.

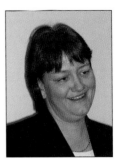

Trust board responsibility

The NHS trust board comprises executive and part-time non-executive board members and has a part-time non-executive chair. The executive directors are usually:

- a chief executive
- a deputy chief executive
- a finance director
- a human resources director
- a medical director
- a nursing director.

Together with the non-executive directors, they share corporate responsibility for all the board's decisions. The board has to ensure that effective executive management arrangements are implemented – the NHS trust board sets the strategic direction of the organization within the overall policies and priorities of the government and the NHS, defining its annual and longer-term objectives and agreeing plans to achieve them.

It also has to monitor the performance of the organization – the NHS trust board oversees the delivery of planned results by monitoring performance against objectives and ensuring corrective action is taken when necessary.

Individually, each executive member of the board has clear and agreed statements of their role and responsibilities and their accountability to the board and, through it, to the public and government offices – in my case, the Welsh Assembly Government.

> the **board** oversees the **delivery** of **planned results**

The director of nursing is the officially designated correspondent and accountable officer for the statutory responsibilities of nursing, associated with the Nursing and Midwifery Order 2001 and all other relevant legislation. He or she provides expert professional advice to the trust board on nursing issues and is responsible for promoting, coordinating and implementing all aspects of the continuous quality improvement agenda.

The role

Requirements

To become an executive director of nursing, you must be a registered general nurse educated to degree level or equivalent and, preferably, have achieved a masters degree. Some organizations also require the individual to have a postregistration qualification in management.

Most postholders will have had a minimum experience of 5 years at a senior nurse level combined with up-to-date knowledge of relevant political and professional issues in healthcare. They will also have evidence of achievement in corporate and clinical leadership within the NHS.

The strategic element

A key part of the role is to lead the strategic direction of nursing within the trust. More often than not, this is achieved within the framework of a trust nursing strategy with objectives that reflect national policy.

This was one of the first objectives addressed when I was appointed as Executive Director of Nursing. My challenge was to create ownership of the strategic vision among the nursing workforce – to get nurses involved in developing the strategy and committed to implementing it. In order, ultimately, to improve the delivery of patient care, the strategy had to be meaningful to frontline nurses, health visitors and midwives.

Overarching themes

In my trust, this is being achieved by addressing six key themes which give an overall view of the areas that have to be addressed by a director of nursing. Education, training and quality are integral to each of these key themes, which are:

- enhancing the patient's experience
- workforce planning
- leadership at all levels
- clinical effectiveness – evidence-based care
- nursing information
- innovation – working in new ways.

Putting policy into practice

As the Director of Nursing, I am also partly responsible for translating the modernization agenda from policy into practice. This about looking at how and who delivers patient care and assessing whether this can be done in a different way – questioning and reviewing what exists, and making evaluated changes. You look specifically at the patient's journey and experience through the healthcare system and identify the need to work in new ways. In partnership with other agencies, you develop and implement new roles that will enhance the quality of patient care.

> you look at the patient's journey and experience

With the ever-increasing need to ensure that patient care is delivered in an effective and efficient manner, the ability to lead in successful change management and practice development is vital to success in the role.

Key skills

To achieve success in both the areas described above, a director of nursing has to:

- have well-developed leadership skills
- be inclusive in his or her approach to implementation
- be able to recognize challenges
- be able to think analytically
- be able to apply effective solutions
- be able to think strategically, while articulating the vision so that it can be implemented with a positive effect on patient care.

Highly developed influencing and communication skills and the ability to demonstrate honesty and integrity throughout are imperative.

Getting there

My career pathway was never really planned but evolved as I moved from one post to the next. Having been appointed as a night sister, it seemed a natural progression to become a ward sister. My decision to become a senior nurse with more of an administrative role rather than being 'hands on' needed a lot more consideration, and I would guess that this would be true for most nurses. Achieving success through others rather than doing it yourself takes some time to learn. I found it difficult to have the level of involvement with patients that I would have ideally liked, although I did try to maintain some kind of daily patient contact. In this role, however, I was able to reflect on intra-professional relationships and develop the expertise in professional protocol and policy needed to ensure safe regulation of the nursing workforce and the duty of care required to safeguard the public.

> achieving **success through others** takes some **time to learn**

My desire to have a wider overview of patient services rather than just patient care eventually took me down the general management route, which provided me with a skills set different from that needed in nursing.

However, the financial skills and business acumen needed for general management are greatly enhanced by the people management, negotiating and influencing skills that are learnt as a nurse. Also, the clinical credibility you have as a nurse should not be underestimated.

The role of deputy director of nursing prepared me for the strategic aspect of the director role. It exposed me to the board process and protocol, but with a safety net (i.e. I wasn't the director!).

On reflection, as I moved through the different roles I gained general professional skills and knowledge, and specific skills in operational management, strategic planning and strategic thinking.

If you are considering working your way to becoming a director of nursing, you need to develop a portfolio of skills, knowledge and attributes. You can start to build these up as you move through different roles in the NHS. All experience is important, and you must draw from it and apply it usefully as you move forward. I could not contribute usefully to organizational objectives if I had not had a breadth of experience in a number of diverse positions within the NHS.

I have always thought that to be a nurse is a privilege. To have the opportunity as a director of nursing to empower and enable nurses, and future nurse leaders, to deliver high standards of patient care and to assist in strengthening and maximizing the contribution of nurses and midwives in delivering the NHS agenda can only confirm that thought.

Voice of experience
The director of nursing

- The patient must always be at the centre of any decision-making
- Working in partnership improves the whole system approach to patient care
- Empower and enable the workforce to deliver effective, innovative and efficient patient-centred care
- You can learn from anyone and everyone and it is your responsibility to develop professionally and personally
- Always see the potential – have belief that it could be achieved and be prepared to help 'make it happen'

education and research

Rosamund Bryar, Professor of Community and Primary Care Nursing and Head of the Public Health and Primary Care Unit, St Bartholomew School of Nursing and Midwifery, City University, London, UK

Today, there are plenty of opportunities in higher education to develop your career as a nurse educator and researcher. Large schools and departments of nursing in universities throughout the country provide pre-registration, postregistration, postgraduate and other education programmes. These departments also have, in many cases, a significant body of

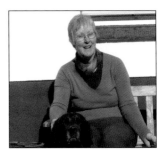

'research active' staff. These include lecturers, senior lecturers, readers and professors who also undertake teaching and other work. Many schools also have research assistants and fellows and members of the academic staff who concentrate on research. Schools of nursing work closely with their local NHS community and many are involved in service development work with their local primary care organizations and hospital trusts.

Integrating teaching, learning and research – elements based in schools and departments – with the promotion of health and the prevention and management of ill health – the business of the NHS – has been something of an ongoing issue between the NHS and the schools and departments of nursing. It is very likely that, in the near future, some healthcare education will move back into the NHS arena

schools of nursing work closely with their local NHS community

and the numbers of nurse educators who also hold service posts in the NHS will increase. The introduction in recent years of the postgraduate teaching diploma or MSc for nurse educators and practice educators opens the way for much more imaginative educational appointments and the possibility that you will be able to move without difficulty between NHS and academic posts. This will mean that you do not need to decide very early on that you want to be a nurse consultant or a professor, as the preparation for both will require you to develop skills in clinical practice, education and research.

Career routes in education

Teaching experience

If you want to have a career in education you need to get as much teaching experience as you can in whatever job you are in. Through this, you will be able to:

- gain experience as a mentor to students and other members of staff
- develop your skills in teaching patients and relatives
- participate in projects that require the development of learning resources for staff or patients
- be a member of your organization's staff training and education committee.

Higher education institutions (HEIs) are always keen to have practitioners teaching on their programmes, so you should approach your local institution with a copy of your CV. You may then want to see if teaching is really for you by applying for a joint appointment in an HEI. Such posts are advertised in the nursing press and also on the website www.jobs.ac.uk.

Teaching qualifications

You will also have to gain a teaching qualification. Initially you may want to gain a qualification as a mentor or practice teacher through taking a short course. Subsequently you may want to qualify as a practice educator/lecturer. Increasingly health service organizations are supporting staff to work for a postgraduate diploma or MSc in education. These provide the individual with a teaching qualification recognized by the

Career destinations – education and research

Nursing and Midwifery Council. Staff with this qualification are then practice educators who provide support to colleagues providing education for healthcare practitioners, as well as being involved in setting and implementing educational strategy in the organization. This qualification also qualifies you as a nurse lecturer and you might then want to apply for a full-time post in an HEI. You can also gain this qualification after you have been appointed in an HEI, as many nursing departments appoint practitioners who are then required to commence the teaching qualification within a number of years of their appointment. As discussed earlier in this chapter, in the future it is probable that there will be many more education posts based in the NHS or joint posts with the NHS, enabling you to maintain and develop your clinical knowledge while at the same time contributing to the education of other healthcare practitioners.

initially you may want to gain a qualification as a mentor or practice teacher

Research and papers

In addition to teaching, nurses who join the academic staff of an HEI as lecturers are usually required to undertake scholarly activity as part of their work. Some lecturers may undertake higher degrees and carry out research as part of their studies. Others gain funding to undertake research. Many universities have internal competitive research awards for staff. Senior lecturers, readers and professors generally undertake a significant amount of research as part of their work. Academic staff who produce four research papers in a 4-year period are deemed 'research active' and the quality of their work is assessed in the research

find out about the research interests of the department you are thinking of applying to

assessment exercise (RAE) that is held approximately every 4 years (the results of the last RAE are available on www.hero.ac.uk/rae). Much of the research in university departments is organized around particular topics or themes to help to produce a coherent body of knowledge, and you should find out about the research interests of the department you are thinking of applying to (for example, by accessing the university website).

Career routes in research and development (R&D)

There are three main R&D career routes: NHS R&D, clinical research and academic study.

NHS R&D

Within NHS trusts and primary care organizations, there are a variety of ways to get involved in research. For example, there are opportunities for secondments to work on projects initiated by other people in the trust. Undertaking a secondment will enable you to establish whether research is for you or if a particular type of research is of interest to you. There are also opportunities to apply for funding for your own project, which may come under a banner of clinical governance or audit. Applying for funding and undertaking such a project will enable you to answer a clinical question that concerns you and will enable you to develop skills such as collecting and presenting data, both of which are fundamental to research practice. The use of a personal development plan will enable you and your manager to recognize your development needs and identify educational courses (e.g. research methods, undergraduate or masters degree programmes) that would develop your research skills (Department of Health 2002).

As your career develops, you may think of working towards becoming a nurse consultant. All nurse consultants are required to participate in research and some may undertake PhDs or professional doctorates (see below). Department of Health guidance on research governance (Department of Health 2001) requires that human resource policies facilitate the development of research skills among NHS staff. This will help you, for example, to become a research nurse, a nurse consultant or a manager who is involved in commissioning research and supporting

> undertaking a **secondment** will enable you to **establish** whether **research is for you**

other staff to develop their research skills. The development of coherent research career pathways is supported by funding from the NHS education contract with HEIs to support nurses to undertake research modules, and undergraduate and higher degrees.

Get to know your R&D office

The majority of NHS organizations have an R&D office and one or more R&D advisors. In addition, many people in NHS organizations have research skills and experience, having undertaken research degrees and research projects. You need to seek out these people and discover what they know and what advice they can give you about resources in your area. In addition, the Internet provides access to a whole range of information (see Table 1).

PhDs and professional doctorates

Some nurses in clinical practice and in management roles in the NHS undertake PhDs at their local university. The choice of supervisor is extremely important and you should thoroughly investigate those that are

Table 1

Useful websites with information on R&D

- **www.dh.gov.uk/policyandguidance/researchanddevelopment/fs/en** provides access to all the latest government R&D information including research awards, workforce capacity building in research and policy documents
- **www.rdlearning.org.uk** provides information on courses, workshops and conferences about research listed under institutions and organizations, making it easy to see what is available in your area
- **www.rdinfo.org.uk** provides extensive up-to-date information on research funding
- **www.rddirect.org.uk** provides information on research and links to many helpful research-related websites
- **www.man.ac.uk/rcn** the Royal College of Nursing (RCN) Research and Development Co-ordinating Centre is an invaluable resource of information on research meetings, jobs, funding and networks

available. Meeting with the higher degrees admissions tutor is also important to understand what the university has to offer and what is expected of you. An increasing number of universities are offering professional doctorates. For these, you need to do a number of interrelated pieces of work concerned with your practice area; some involve attending taught courses. If you want to develop your practice at doctoral level and develop your research skills, but you do not intend to be a full-time researcher, then it is worth considering undertaking a professional doctorate rather than a PhD.

an **increasing number** of **universities** are offering a **professional doctorate**

Clinical research

Many nurses are employed in the NHS and in companies, for example, in pharmaceutical companies, as clinical research nurses who are involved in clinical trials of new drugs and other treatments. Nurses in these posts coordinate the recruitment of patients and manage the process of the trial and collection of data, for example, in the form of specimens. This type of research allows for continued involvement with patients and the use of a wide range of nursing skills. Nurses in these posts have a need for continuing professional development and career development in their chosen area; further information about this is provided by the RCN at www.man.ac.uk/rcn/clinresgrades.htm.

Academic study

Within universities, nurses may become contract researchers undertaking research as their main activity or they may become lecturers undertaking research as part of their role. Universities advertise these posts in the press, through the RCN Co-ordinating Centre and on the Internet at www.jobs.ac.uk. The contracts, for contract researchers, are generally for 1–3 years and some enable people to register for higher degrees. Contract researchers are generally involved in the day-to-day management of projects and in producing new research bids to fund their next period of employment. There is also the opportunity for career progression from research assistant to senior research fellow. Other nurses join the academic staff as lecturers and, as described above, may then become involved in research activity.

Becoming a professor

You might feel that you want to go all the way, and set your sights on a Chair in nursing. Up to now, the most usual way for a person to become a professor in nursing has been through following a research career. To become a professor, you have to demonstrate that you meet criteria that are equivalent for all professors in the university. For example, you have to demonstrate that:

- you have undertaken research in a coherent area of practice, theory or method
- you have obtained research funding for your research
- you have published in academic journals and presented your findings to peers at conferences.

Teaching experience or administrative and management skills may be required for some appointments, but the key criteria to date have focused on the contribution of the person to research. So an individual might gain a PhD and then work his or her way to be a professor through a number of appointments as a researcher, then lecturer, senior lecturer and reader – all the time continuing to develop and extend their research experience until appointed through internal promotion or application to another institution as a professor.

I should say, at this point, that my career route has been slightly different: the first time I thought seriously about becoming a professor was only 2 years before I became one! In my career, I have moved back and forth between practice and academic settings and I took an opportunistic rather than a planned approach to becoming a professor. This has suited me because, throughout my career, I have valued being able to have a 'foot in both camps': the NHS and universities.

> I have **valued** being able to have a **'foot** in **both camps':** the NHS and **universities**

The unit in which I now work is involved in education, research and practice development activities with local primary care trusts in East

London. Staff in the unit contribute to pre-registration and postregistration teaching up to PhD level; they undertake research locally and at national and international levels in collaboration with colleagues in other universities. They also work with colleagues in the local primary care trusts on service development activities – these lead to real change in practice and service organization. Several staff in the unit hold joint appointments in the NHS and I am a non-executive director of City and Hackney Teaching Primary Care Trust. The aim is to have current insight into issues in the NHS and the academic world. Our higher education knowledge can then be used to inform our NHS activities and our NHS involvement can be used to inform research and teaching in the higher education institutions.

Working with practitioners and managers in the NHS in supporting practice change and development has given me (and continues to give me) the greatest satisfaction. In my present post, I value being able to influence the development of nursing programmes so that they have a greater focus on primary care and public health. I enjoy being able to participate in research with other colleagues, though I continually feel as though I do not have enough time for this! I enjoy supervising research students and seeing them and their work develop over the period of their registration. As our service and practice development work expands, it is rewarding to see the way colleagues in the unit have contributed to changes in practice and the way that new, longer-term projects build on each other. In my present role, the thing that is brought home to me over and over again is the value of integrating practice, education and research in developing practice, informing teaching and in raising research questions.

> ## supporting practice change and development has given me the greatest satisfaction

Nurses in research – the future

Striving towards evidence-based practice is essential to help ensure nurses and other healthcare practitioners provide the best possible care (Bryar and Griffiths, 2003). Organizations such as the Healthcare Commission and the National Institute for Clinical Excellence (NICE) have been put in place to monitor healthcare standards and to produce guidelines based on current evidence. Research is needed in all areas of clinical practice to provide the evidence on which to base best practice; more nurses, midwives and health visitors with experience of research are going to be needed for this. And more practitioners with facilitation and implementation skills are going to be needed to support staff in changing their practice, as the translation of research findings into practice is extremely challenging.

Voice of experience
The professor

- Practice and develop your teaching skills in whatever job you are in
- Make contact with the educational leaders in your organization and ensure that they are aware of your interest in education
- Find people active in research and research networks in your local area to provide you with support
- Seek out a mentor or leader in education or research and development who can provide you with guidance and encouragement
- Make contact with the nurse educators in your local higher education institution
- Work with others to develop research ideas, as collaborative research develops your knowledge and provides a range of partners who can make different contributions to the research process
- Map out a career pathway to your Chair to enable you to make the right decisions along the way

Further reading

Bryar RM, Griffiths JM, eds. *Practice Development in Community Nursing. Principles and Processes.* London: Arnold, 2003.

Department of Health. *Research Governance Framework for Health and Social Care.* London: TSO, 2001.

Department of Health. Funding Learning and Development for the Healthcare Workforce. *Consultation on the Review of NHS Education and Training Funding and the Review of Contract Benchmarking for NHS Funded Education and Training.* London: Department of Health, 2002.

Royal College of Nursing. *The Clinical Research Nurse in NHS Trusts and GP Practices: Guidance for Nurses and their Employers.* RCN Employment Brief 22/98 (available from www.man.ac.uk/rcn/clinresgrades.htm).

chief executive of a trust

Mark Morgan, Chief Executive of Rushcliffe Primary
Care Trust, Nottingham, UK

I became the Chief Executive of Rushcliffe Primary Care Trust in 2001, having started out in the NHS as a registered mental health nurse. Being a chief executive is hard work but potentially very rewarding. My background as a nurse has proven invaluable and, as I describe later, nurses generally have qualities and skills that can serve them well in managerial positions such as chief executive. Such positions offer nurses ways to improve patient care in exciting and rewarding ways.

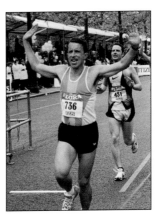

The role of chief executive

The chief executive of an NHS trust sits on the board of that trust alongside other executive and non-executive directors. There is a requirement for a non-executive chair, a director of finance, a medical director (or a director of public health and a professional executive committee [PEC] chair in primary care trusts [PCTs]), and a director of nursing. In addition, there must be an equal balance between executive and non-executive directors, with the chair holding the casting vote.

> nurses generally have qualities and skills that can serve them well in managerial positions

The chief executive has four key areas of responsibility, and these are described below.

Managing the organization's performance

The chief executive has the overall management responsibility for the effective performance of the organization. This means he or she is accountable for more than 400 NHS targets (plus the others that apply to all businesses, such as health and safety, fire, and European law).

The government feels that measuring performance against planned NHS targets is key to maintaining public confidence in the NHS. This is part of the relentless drive for improvement. At one level, this means getting more out of the resources that we currently employ (historically, the NHS has done this by working people harder). At the same time, virtually everybody in and around the NHS, including government ministers, recognizes that we will not deliver the government's 10-year agenda for the NHS unless there is a radical rethink of how services are delivered. Chief executives are accountable for both areas of work and, as part of this, we have to engage our staff in redesigning the service and the way in which they work.

> we have to **engage** our **staff** in **redesigning** the **service**

Accountability for expenditure

The chief executive is the 'accountable officer', which means that he or she is accountable to Parliament for the expenditure of taxpayers' money. In reality, this doesn't mean making a regular trip to Parliament, but that you're exposed to a series of scrutiny bodies (such as external auditors). These require signed assurances of key pieces of work for which internal systems must be in place – an example is the preparation of waiting-list information. The auditors can demand to examine these processes to ensure that your organization is acting correctly. Unfairly, some people think this is a paper exercise, but a read through of the health press should quickly dispel any doubts – of the 12 trusts given 'no stars' in the 2001 performance rating system, only one had the same chief executive one year later!

Rigorous systems need to be in place to take these duties forward. These systems are subject to external scrutiny by bodies such as the Healthcare Commission in England (formerly the Commission for Health Improvement). When I was the director of nursing of a trust with lead responsibility for clinical governance, we had a fairly heated discussion about these statutory duties. One position put forward was that they were less important than the financial duties. The chief executive could override the quality duty, it was argued, in order to meet the financial ones. It is only now, with the impact of the clinical governance reviews, that we know how wrong this thinking was.

Leading the organization and senior team

Chief executives are responsible for setting the tone of the organization and, along with the lay chairs, we are the external face to politicians and to leaders in the statutory and voluntary sectors. There is currently a large emphasis on the leaders of organizations. While this has included a focus on clinical leaders, it is the managerial leaders who are consistently scrutinized. When reports from independent enquiries criticize poor organizational culture, it is to the NHS board that the public

> chief executives are responsible for setting the tone of the organization

and the wider NHS look for accountability. It is the role of managerial leaders to develop leadership throughout the organization and in all staff. The responsibility for any absence of such leadership is frequently laid at the door of one person, the chief executive.

Becoming a chief executive

I ended up in the NHS by accident. I intended to do a science-based course at university and then follow this with some career or other. After a spell doing some voluntary work on a ward for older people in the final stages of dementia, I took up the role of nursing assistant. I was lucky to work with some inspirational colleagues who encouraged me to apply for nursing training and my science course was history!

My own career 'journey' (Table 1) has been practically oriented and training-based. And while the world that is the NHS is changing all the time, the sort of route I followed remains as viable today as it was when I first set out on it – the key is to keep ahead of developments and to assume that change is inevitable. This, in my view, helps you to remain professionally adaptable.

The list in Table 1 emphasizes how I changed roles to develop new skills. Whenever I move to a new role, I rigorously assess the transferable skills that I can take with me. Formal assessment using management competency frameworks, as well as more personality-based preferences, are increasingly used in recruitment to more senior positions. I advise you to do some of these in your own time, well ahead of possible career movements, so that you are absolutely clear about your own strengths and weaknesses.

But it's also important to realize that the skills we learn early on in our working lives stay with us. Personally, there are many dimensions of my early nursing work that I still find relevant today. While these are not unique to nurses, they are often characteristic. For example, nursing experience tends to:

- make you think first and foremost about patients
- mean you can work with others without having to control them

Table 1

My personal pathway to chief executive

1982	Trained as registered mental nurse
1988	Community psychiatric nurse
1991	Community services manager
1993	Directorate manager, mental health
1995	Clinical director, learning disabilities
1998	Director of nursing
2001	Chief executive

- mean you've had opportunities to lead large 24-hour teams early on in your management career
- make you feel comfortable sharing success with a much wider team, while knowing that your contribution has been vital
- mean that you have a 'can do' attitude – if a job has to be done, you'll get on and do it.

For these reasons, you can have significant advantages over some of your colleagues in management roles.

Competencies for the role

On election, the Labour administration in England committed itself to establishing a new NHS organization – the primary care trust (PCT) – which was required to take the leading role in changing the NHS. Recognizing that leadership would be critical in these new organizations, the Department of Health commissioned Hay Consulting to develop a competency framework for PCT chief executives (Table 2). You'll see that few competencies are specific to the work of a PCT but instead they apply to most NHS chief executive roles.

For me, many of the competencies I am expected to demonstrate have been areas of ongoing development throughout my NHS career: working across disciplines and agencies, getting things done by influence rather than control, and putting patients at the heart of what we do when planning and delivering services.

In addition to the formal competencies, you need:
- humility
- strong values and an ability to retain perspective on why we are really here
- resilience and the ability to learn from difficult situations
- the ability to manage a fairly high level of pressure, preferably by having other balancing interests
- to be comfortable with uncertainty and able to tolerate personal uncertainty (turnover at chief executive level can be quite high).

Effective learning is key

One of the things I've retained from early management courses is a profile of my learning styles. This simple questionnaire gives you a formal but

Table 2

Leadership competencies of a PCT chief executive*

Personal competencies
- Lead others with vision, passion and pride
- Get things done by being focused and resourceful
- Build bonds through collaboration and understanding
- Maintain commitment by strength and determination
- Work with others by building support and respect

Technical competencies
- Provide leadership for the trust
- Ensure that national and local agendas are delivered
- Work with partners to serve the healthcare needs of the local community
- Represent the trust to the public
- Provide a corporate governance structure in keeping with the principles and standards set out by the Department of Health
- Account for the trust's performance to the board
- Enable staff to make a contribution to the trust
- Manage the performance of the trust's staff
- Manage the trust's resources

*From: Department of Health. *A Competency Framework for PCT Leadership.* London: TSO, 2002

broadly structured way of focusing on how you learn best. For some of us, it may mean we need to practise doing something before we fully learn how to exercise a new skill. Others among us need to understand the theory or reasons why we would need to have this skill and how we would need to use it. While it is important to make best use of our learning style to learn efficiently, such approaches are preferences only and complementing them with other styles is very helpful. A personal example is that, despite having a preference for more experiential development programmes, I decided to do a masters degree in business administration (an MBA). I recognized that such a qualification was considered an essential prerequisite for many top management posts (but like a first degree, many qualifications can get you to the interview stage of top posts but they don't get you the job – that's down to you and the panel!).

One of the stereotypes around nurses as managers is that they're less comfortable with specialist areas such as human resources, finance and planning. While I found these areas challenging, many of these subjects come down to technical approaches that have to be learnt, not instinctive abilities. For me, the MBA was important in developing these skills and the confidence that went with them.

Moving outside the comfort zone

If you're thinking about a career in management you might also want to consider looking for opportunities to work in areas you're less familiar with. For example, I moved from rehabilitation psychiatry to acute psychiatry, from mental health to learning disability, from general management to nursing, and from nursing to chief executive. You're staying outside your comfort zone and seeking to broaden your understanding and skill base in this hugely diverse and complex world of healthcare.

Learning from experience

Most experiences can be a source of learning. As a student nurse, I saw an example of ill treatment of a client. The feelings I had about how this was managed still influence my thinking on such issues today. When I worked as a community psychiatric nurse, I had some difficulties with a manager. I raised my perception of our differences, and we used our discussions as a way of developing a much stronger working relationship. Later in my career I adopted this same approach and this reinforced to me the importance of learning from experiences (even the difficult ones) all the time.

When I became a manager, I worked for some time in an area with very poor industrial relations. Disciplinary processes were often used and the hearings adversarial and acrimonious. Despite the personal discomfort I felt at having to work in such an environment, it led me to recognize the enormous importance that has to be placed on the process associated with discipline and grievance. In a later role, I had to take extremely difficult decisions about terminating staff employment and referring individual cases for police action. Previous mistakes that I'd made, and clarity about the importance of preliminary work, enabled me to make a much more just series of decisions.

What it's really like

For me, some aspects of the role have been significantly less stressful than I anticipated. Often you hear that life in one of these roles is lonely. Usually people mean that, ultimately, there's no one to turn to for helpful advice. This has not (yet!) been the case for me. Throughout my career I've been fortunate to develop and maintain a group of close colleagues in or near the organizations in which I've worked. These have often been as, if not more, helpful than any particular line manager. Moving from being an executive director to a chief executive did not feel unduly stressful because I could still rely on this close group and use them as a sounding board for the more difficult issues that have arisen.

> some aspects of the role have been significantly less stressful than anticipated

Professional relationships

Chief executives of NHS trusts have a senior management team that includes some clinically trained staff (such as the medical director and nursing director). They then have a board. PCTs on the other hand have a professional executive committee (PEC) in addition to the board. The PEC comprises a combination of credible (and still practising) senior clinical staff and senior managers and it is the place where clinical priorities and strategies are agreed and developed.

The chief executive who is a nurse will, nevertheless, have a senior nurse whose role it is to provide the guidance the chief executive needs on key issues. It is crucial that you don't mix the roles – you have to be guided by what your senior nurse tells you rather than resorting to your own experience or perspectives. There is no reason to challenge (or support) the advice given to you by the director of nursing any more or less than any other corporate director.

This ability to work with a range of senior professionals, each with a strong contribution (often personality) and significant drive, is a real challenge. It is, nevertheless, key to success. No matter how strong or capable a chief executive, a weak team (at either the executive or the non-executive level) means the organization is destined to fail. From the very start of your career in nursing, you can start to think about which teams work well, and why, and you can draw on this later when you start to build your own teams.

start to **think** about **which teams work well,** and **why**

The pressures

Unsurprisingly, there are pressures on a chief executive. PCTs, for example, are new organizations with high political expectations placed on them. They have a much wider set of responsibilities and less management resources than trusts. In the end, this can take a toll on the whole team. As the chief executive, it is up to you to ensure that your team can cope with reasonable demands and to shelter them from any unreasonable expectations.

Another less palatable aspect of being a chief executive is that you work long hours. Not only do you have to put in the hours to achieve what's expected, but you also have to accommodate the working patterns of those with whom you collaborate. For example, meetings with GPs are generally held in the evenings, and it can sometimes be hard to meet domestic commitments. In my case, I find myself working late on at least one evening a week.

Maintaining professional registration

Finally, it is worth mentioning how nurses working in non-nursing roles maintain professional registration – the Nursing and Midwifery Council is clear that this is crucial. Maintaining professional registration is very challenging. Whilst much of my work is, I believe, informed by my nursing registration, the role of chief executive is not one that maintains your ability to practice. The Nursing and Midwifery Council has, I understand, given some thought to this but more guidance is needed.

- Stay adaptable and recognize and develop transferable skills
- Seize opportunities, even if they seem daunting at first
- Learn from and reflect on everything you encounter
- Use your judgment and intuition, but be prepared to learn from the times when these turn out to be wrong
- Recognize what motivates you at work

A typical day

I tend to arrive at work at about 7.30 am and work through until 6 pm. On one and sometimes two evenings a week I have an evening meeting but I then try to have at least a little time away from the office rather than work straight through. Much of my working day is spent in meetings and approximately one-third concern the internal workings of my PCT and the other two-thirds the external relationship between my organization and other local healthcare organizations. Locally my board and the strategic health authority expect chief executives to lead on key work across the health community. Some of my responsibilities have included leading the financial and commercial closure of a public/private partnership to replace primary care premises locally, and the same for the establishment of an independent sector treatment centre locally.

The future of the chief executive

New policies (such as practice-based commissioning) are being discussed by politicians, and the political parties are airing their views about the role of administration/management (delete as you see fit!). Unsurprisingly, I believe that as NHS spending approaches over £100 billion per year the taxpayer has a right to know that it is being spent well and is tightly monitored. PCTs, with their role of driving forward on public health and a primary-care-led NHS, will certainly have a role in some shape or form.

Personally, I've really enjoyed establishing a new organization and leading it to some early successes. I relish the challenges involved in taking it to a new phase, to embed a culture of patients, clinicians, and managers working together as a powerful force for change. My background as a nurse has been truly invaluable and it remains something of which I am extremely proud.

Further reading

Collins J. Level 5 Leadership. *Harvard Business Review* 2001 (Jan).

Department of Health. *The New NHS: Modern, Dependable.* London: HMSO, 1997.

Department of Health. *Patient and Public Involvement in the New NHS.* London: TSO, 2003.

Department of Health. *Shifting the Balance of Power: The Next Steps.* London: TSO, 2002.

Goldman D. Leadership That Gets Results. *Harvard Business Review* 2002 (March).

Honey P, Mumford A. *Using Your Learning Styles,* 3rd edn. Maidenhead: Peter Honey Publications, 1995.

NHS Executive. *PCTs: Establishing Better Services.* London: TSO, 1999.

audit and inspection

Maureen Burton, Operations Project Manager,
Healthcare Commission

Think about a rollercoaster ride at a theme park. As you wait anxiously for your turn, you can hear the screams in the distance ... maybe it's excitement, maybe it's fear, maybe anticipation, or maybe it's all of these. You can see some of the ride but not the whole construction, just bits that you try to piece together. You move slowly along with some trepidation and reach the front of the queue. You climb on board, you sit down, the bar comes down and there's no turning back. You are

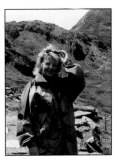

sitting in the carriage and it crawls along slowly, you can hear the ratchet beside you clicking as it pulls you slowly up, up and up you go, click, click, click. You reach the top and you can't see, you pause, take a deep breath, absolutely no turning back now and then whoosh, you drop at speed. You come to a bend, turn left, turn right and spin around and this keeps on going, becoming a bit of a blur. You then enter a black tunnel, you slow down and just when you think it's all over, you drop down again, more turning and spinning. Just as you're getting used to it you stop, the bar is lifted and you feel exhilarated, excited or exhausted and probably all three, but know that if you are going to conquer the rollercoaster you will have to do it all again.

think about
a rollercoaster ride at a
theme park ...

That sums up how I felt when I first started working for a national organization aimed at reviewing and inspecting healthcare, the Commission for Health Improvement (the predecessor of the Healthcare Commission). Read on ...

The Healthcare Commission

The Healthcare Commission was established in April 2004 to promote improvement in the quality of NHS and independent healthcare across England and Wales. It not only replaced the Commission for Health Improvement, but took over the private and voluntary healthcare functions of the National Care Standards Commission and the functions of the Audit Commission with respect to national studies of efficiency, effectiveness and economy of healthcare. The Healthcare Commission provides independent assessment of the standards of services, whether they are provided by the NHS, private healthcare or voluntary organizations, and reports on the quality of healthcare and value for money offered by all healthcare organizations. It also licenses private and voluntary healthcare establishments, investigates serious failures in healthcare, reviews data quality relating to healthcare and administers the second stage of the NHS complaints process. The Healthcare Commission aims to promote the coordination of reviews, inspections and assessments of healthcare undertaken by other bodies and in doing so reduce the overall burden of scrutiny of healthcare for individual organizations.

> the Healthcare Commission provides independent assessment of the standards

Learning from experience

One of my first experiences was to help another review manager in an organization that had, only the weekend before, provided the headlines in the local newspapers. The articles had been very critical of some of the services provided. I had expected to observe the process only, but one of the reviewers became ill and I took over a number of interviews. One of the first lessons I learnt was 'always be prepared to get involved'. My emotions were significantly tested when I went to support another colleague holding interviews with local people about their hospital services. I will never forget the story related by a man about his mother and her experience of care in the last 3 months of her life. It was a traumatic story of neglect, poor communication, a lack of information and a family left devastated by their experiences of the NHS. At the end

Career destinations – audit and inspection

of his story, the man got up and abruptly left – it seemed too painful to remain any longer. The purpose of sharing his family's experiences was so that another family could be spared such an episode. I turned to my colleague, tears streaming down both our faces, both of us feeling ashamed and angry at the account of rude and dismissive attitudes. My next lesson was to be prepared for whatever or whomsoever walked through the door with their personal story. My resolve was strengthened by this experience and the values of an organization setting out to make real improvements for patients, service users and carers reinforced.

Not all the stories are as traumatizing – many are inspiring. I cannot forget the man who, half way through an interview, pulled open his shirt to show me the scar from his recent heart operation and what a zest for life he had, or the person who had felt life had nothing to offer, arms scarred mercilessly through self-abuse, finding support and care to plan and have a future. The role of review manager provided opportunities to meet with individual staff, to listen to their personal contributions to the services and share their passions, hopes and fears for the health service to which they are committed.

Moving into the area

Nurses joining the Healthcare Commission can expect to be involved in a challenging and changing environment as healthcare standards and systems of assessment develop. Nurses have often taken and set the lead for developing services and ensuring that they meet the needs of individual patients, service users, their relatives and carers – joining a national body like the Healthcare Commission is a great opportunity to extend this role. The Commission's values are to focus on positive outcomes for patients, users of services and the public. It works in partnership with others and provides independent and fair assessment and review. Through the Commission, individuals can contribute to developing and improving standards within individual healthcare organizations and for NHS and independent healthcare at a national level.

> nurses have often taken and set the lead for developing services

My initial role was as a review manager, which meant taking the lead in managing clinical governance reviews (reviewing clinical governance arrangements within individual organizations and how these impacted directly on care and services for patients, service users and carers). This opened a whole new world to me. I was working alongside colleagues who collated and analysed data and information, strategists and policy makers, politicians and national leaders in clinical and service development and teams of communications experts who liaised with the public and media. But this was balanced with the direct contact I retained with those who provided and received services.

Seeing the 'big picture'

For a career in healthcare assessment, investigation and review, I'd say you need to be able to see the 'big picture', understand the political environment in which healthcare operates and believe in the value of continuous improvement. It's essential to have a good knowledge of the NHS and its associated stakeholders, and the structure of healthcare delivery in the UK. You also need the desire to improve care and services for patients, service users and carers. Working in this type of role gives you an opportunity to develop analytical skills, to analyse complex quantitative and qualitative data and to develop further your communication skills, as you'll be involved in preparing formal reports and making presentations. The benefits are that you contribute to projects, reviews and inspections that really make a difference to people's lives.

> you need to believe in the value of continuous improvement

A different way of working

You also need to be able to work in a flexible way, not spending so much time at your office base as you may have in previous roles. Working nationally, I can be at venues and locations throughout the country and often it is most convenient to work from home. This requires a different approach to the organization and planning of work commitments and responsibilities to ensure an effective and achievable work/life balance. At times, working in the evenings and at weekends will be essential to meet critical deadlines and will form part of the overall work pattern. Also, you may work within a team that you will not necessarily see face to face on a regular basis. This takes a bit more effort to ensure that communication is effective and it makes corporate days and team meetings priorities in the diary. With a laptop and mobile phone, you can work anywhere, and the need to develop competent computer skills is paramount. Developing these new ways of working to meet the given timeframes and parameters requires the ability to adapt and change to suit the circumstances of each project. This, in turn, provides, for me, a stimulating, varied and interesting work life.

Acting professionally

You also need to be able to suspend judgment and employ tact, diplomacy and professionalism in all situations. You need to remember that all statements, assessments and conclusions need to be backed by sufficient evidence. Other personal qualities you need include the ability to work effectively within a team, and to be able to challenge and be challenged on anything and everything. In return, the opportunity to work with a variety of highly committed people who see the world from different perspectives is both demanding and enlightening. Like the rollercoaster ride, it is sometimes uncomfortable, sometimes scary and painful, but always exciting and exhilarating, with never a dull moment.

All change!

Being part of a national organization that then merges with other review and inspection bodies (as happened when the Commission for Health Improvement became part of the Commission for Healthcare, Audit and Inspection) offers more opportunities and challenges. Working in a high-profile organization like this does not mean that you are immune from the regular re-organizations and changes that occur throughout the NHS at all levels. So just when you are feeling reasonably comfortable

when **change happens, reflect back** on **what you've learnt** with your role and responsibilities, everything changes. One of the lessons that I learnt early on in my career is that, when change happens, you should reflect back on what you've learnt, how you've grown, and what areas you've become competent in and take those with you to the next role and challenge. Change also provides opportunities to leave behind all the ways of working that you've not valued.

With the growth and development of a young organization, opportunities arise. I have found myself contributing to the development of methods and systems of assessment as well as inspections, reviews and investigations. On the downside, as with many jobs, the schedules can be exhausting and often involve travel away from home. Understanding and strong personal support are essential.

Tips for success

I've had a varied and enjoyable nursing career to date. With every role, every responsibility, every training and development programme, I can now see I was building a portfolio of skills that would help in successive roles and in my current role as an operations project manager with the Healthcare Commission. There are a few key lessons that I'd like to share.

Get your studying done early

I carried on studying part-time throughout my nursing career, and always tried to consider what additional training or development opportunity would improve my knowledge, skills and competence. I was fortunate that my employers always supported my ambitions. Looking back, I can see how important it was to get as much of the study completed before I found myself in a senior role. It would be more difficult in my current role, for instance, to attend any regular off-the-job training, as this would cut into the planned programmes I manage and it would also restrict the flexibility I need to meet key people with very full schedules.

Jump at opportunities

The proud day I qualified as a staff nurse, I was asked what I wanted to do next. I remember replying, without hesitation, that I wanted to be the ward sister. The opportunity of becoming a sister within a psychiatric unit came within a year. It was probably rather soon to take on such a responsibility, but it made me value and rely on the support, advice and guidance of a number of colleagues and it taught me the essential importance of being able to work effectively as part of a team. On balance though, I would still recommend to anyone that if a selection panel considers that you are ready, jump at the opportunity for an early test of your abilities. At the time, I thought about my reasons for taking on this more senior nursing role carefully. I knew that it definitely wasn't about being in charge, nor was it about status or increased responsibility. I really wanted to be in a position to influence care standards and the ways that these could and should be delivered. The ability to positively impact on the lives of others and create positive working environments became a driving force in my career.

Broaden your experiences

I would recommend gaining experience in both acute care and community settings if you want to move into a strategic role. I did the certificate course in community psychiatric nursing, and found that it provided opportunities to train and work with an array of health, social care and education colleagues. It also gave me an appreciation of the need to understand the environment in which individuals live, the obstacles sometimes faced through family history and the differing personal, cultural and spiritual needs of individuals and groups within society.

A word about being inspected

From my experience of being the 'inspector', a number of recurring issues for those being inspected have arisen – I would like to pass on some of these to any of you who may find yourself in this position.

Working to specified high standards, and developing care pathways and policies based on the best evidence and research available

when the 'inspectors' call you really do need to be prepared

Voice of experience

The audit and inspection professional

- Complete as much part-time study as possible early on (before you find yourself in a senior role)
- If you find yourself a nurse in a management role, get some management development
- Taking sideways moves often creates new career development opportunities
- Have confidence in your abilities and don't be shy about sharing your ambitions with people who can help you realize them
- Seek opportunities to work in different settings. If you see opportunities to work at a different level (e.g. within a trust, strategic health authority or nationally), give it serious consideration – the NHS is a complex system and seeing how the pieces fit together is increasingly important
- If you get involved in quality improvement and hear about very poor services, it will be painful for you as well as the service user and you need to be ready to cope with these feelings
- Regularly reflect on what you have learnt, how you have grown, and the areas in which you have become competent
- Make and take opportunities for learning wherever possible and, in particular, develop skills in audit and research
- Make sure that if you make assessments or reach conclusions, you have evidence to support your evaluation

are now an integral part of healthcare management. In everyday nursing, nurses need to develop and use their audit and research skills to critically appraise and audit standards and ways of working, particularly across multidisciplinary team working. However, when the 'inspectors' call you really do need to be prepared and able to demonstrate clearly how standards are set, implemented, audited and re-audited. Some organizations I've visited have very recently approved a paper that has proposed how this work would be undertaken – it soon becomes apparent if the ink is still wet!

Any actions arising from audit and review need to state clear and measurable outcomes, with progress and achievement regularly monitored. Often the proposed outcomes are simply further actions – it is critical that the outcomes relate to quantifiable improvements. Reviewing standards needs to be built into a constant cycle and is a fundamental part of team working. External review, audit and inspection can be viewed either as something to be feared or as something to help improve and develop practice, providing an opportunity to learn from mistakes and share good practice. Just like those of you who provide and deliver services, external reviewers and inspectors have the needs of patients, service users and the public at the heart of what they do. Being open and honest about what has been developed and what works well, and highlighting concerns or issues to be addressed will help lead to positive relationships so that we can work together to improve the quality of care.

Further reading

Department of Health. *National Standards, Local Action. Health and Social Care Standards and Planning Framework 2005/6–2007/8.* TSO: London, 2004 (available from www.dh.gov.uk/publications).

inside a government department

Tina Donnelly, former Nursing Officer, Welsh Assembly Government, and currently Director of the Royal College of Nursing in Wales

Working as a nurse in a government department is a tremendously rewarding role, and offers the postholder the chance to inform and shape policy that will affect nurses and nursing throughout the UK. The ultimate goal of any professional health advisor working as a civil servant is to promote health and develop health policies that will improve care in the NHS and the independent sector.

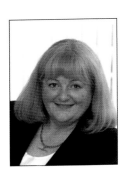

Nurses within government departments can work in a variety of roles, either on secondment or in substantive positions as civil servants or nursing officers. A nurse who is seconded to work in a government department is usually required to perform a specific role/task for a fixed term and remains on his or her currently held terms and conditions of employment. This may mean being employed to project manage an important area of work – an example being to lead on the production of a strategy document which draws on the specialist professional skills of the individual nurse who undertakes the secondment. A nursing officer is normally a substantive position and the postholder has civil service terms and conditions of employment. A nursing officer is professionally accountable directly to the chief nursing officer.

the **ultimate goal** is to **promote health**

The government requires contemporary, expert professional advice. For nurses who can meet the requirements, there are fixed-term appointments as consultants, advisors and secondees. Their job titles usually reflect their role – for example, 'project manager research strategy' for a nurse who is project managing the drafting and consultation of a nursing research strategy. These positions may be full-time or part-time. Alternatively, some nurses are released from their primary positions to undertake specific roles, either taking the place of permanent employees or 'gap-filling' vacancies to ensure that the work of substantive posts continues until they can be filled through the normal recruitment procedures. There is also the opportunity to undertake project work as a nurse researcher.

> the **government** requires **contemporary, expert professional advice**

Nursing officers

Government health departments have devolved responsibility for the delivery of health and social services in England, Wales, Scotland and Northern Ireland. Each health department has a chief nursing officer who has accountability for formulating and advising on all aspects of nursing, midwifery and health-visiting policy. The chief nursing officer is supported by a team of nursing officers and also by 'career civil servants', who have a supportive administrative role.

Nursing officers are senior nurses with a high level of expertise in the area for which they have the lead advisory role. In almost all cases, they are professionally accountable to the chief nursing officer, and provide expert advice to him or her, the minister for health, other politicians and to civil service government officials. Often nursing officers have the opportunities to lead on key challenges and to take nurses and nursing forward into the next decade and beyond.

To become a nursing officer, you need to be a registered nurse and to have undergone postregistration training. You also need to have experience of operating at senior level. Often the minimum educational requirement is a masters degree. You will also need the ability to engage with a wide network of professional staff working within the healthcare community – you will be expected to consult regularly with them when seeking to develop policy that will impact on service delivery to patients. You will probably have to demonstrate your experience of having done this in the past. It's important to have live registration with the Nursing and Midwifery Council, as you are accountable for the professional advice you give as a nursing officer. The remits of nursing officers vary within each of the government departments in terms of the role assigned. Sometimes they are supported by experienced nurses seconded into the department to offer expert clinical advice in support of specific policy initiatives.

In my role as a nursing officer, I was employed on a permanent basis in the Welsh Assembly Government. I provided advice to the National Assembly for Wales, the Welsh Assembly Government, the Chief Nursing Officer for Wales and civil service colleagues. My remit was to provide specialist advice on:

- the training and education of pre-registration and postregistration nurses, midwives and health visitors
- the research and development agenda in nursing
- the regulation of nurses, midwives and health visitors
- nurse leadership
- human resources.

Experience

As a nursing officer, it's important to have a track record of appropriate and specific experience of the areas in which you will be required to work. But it's also essential to have broad-based experience in nursing, as the more experience you have, the better informed you are and this makes you a lot more confident in your role. It also goes a long way to establishing your credibility among other advisors and colleagues.

For my role, it was essential that I was an experienced researcher with a history of engaging in research, teaching research methods and evaluating research findings (since research underpins all areas of practice and education). It was also useful to have had experience in commissioning research and participating as a member of an academic scrutiny panel that, among other things, considered the ethical implications of research.

In terms of providing advice on the commissioning of education and training of nurses, midwives and health visitors and in formulating policies to advance the nursing professions, it was essential that I was a qualified nurse teacher and had experience in this area. While I did train as a midwife (in the late 1970s), the contemporary advice for midwifery and health-visiting practice that I used to inform my role in commissioning training places was provided by other nursing officers whose remits covered these areas.

Problem-solving abilities

The skills required to be a nursing officer centre on relevant experience and training. Nursing officers have to analyse complex problems, argue points logically and propose workable recommendations supported by evidence. You need to be able see both sides of the argument, as you have to reach a balanced view. I found that my nursing background helped me to become an expert problem solver – assessing patients' needs and then creating care plans based on research evidence while ensuring that they also encompassed patients' wishes is good preparation. Working within an ever-changing NHS also offers opportunities to develop your imagination, creativity and resourcefulness in developing and implementing new policies. Build on these opportunities as, once you are a nursing officer, you'll be expected to use your experience to produce or propose:

- constructive ideas
- practical solutions
- workable actions plans.

Communication skills

Nursing officers need excellent communication skills – written and oral. You need to be able to write clearly, concisely and logically across a range of government and nursing business, while adapting a style and tone that keeps the needs of the recipient uppermost. The skill of speaking lucidly while keeping to the point comes with experience. You also need to be able to discuss, argue and defend a point of view while recognizing the weight of counter-arguments. As a nurse, you sometimes have to be an advocate, striving to get what is best for the patient – developing your communication skills in times such as these will stand you in good stead.

As a nursing officer, you'll also need to make speeches and give presentations in a variety of settings, with the audience ranging from small committees to large government bodies and agencies. In my case, because my remit encompassed regulation, I also made presentations to colleagues in other government departments and, on occasions, the regulatory body. From time to time, you are also going to have to express independent and unwelcome opinions to strong-minded and sometimes senior colleagues across the healthcare spectrum, within your own country and to colleagues in other countries. You need to be comfortable with this – you'll need to support your decisions with confidence, and be assertive and persuasive.

the skill of speaking lucidly while keeping to the point comes with experience

Project management

If you get the chance to develop your project management skills, take it. It's very useful to have learnt and developed techniques and methods of keeping things on track, particularly if you have several projects running at the same time.

Personal strengths

Working in government is achievement-oriented – managing your own work within tight deadlines requires energy and commitment. You need to believe in what you are doing, and that the overall aim is to benefit the patient/client, and their families. To work in the civil service, you need to be productive, reliable under pressure and adaptable in the face of change. The nursing officer role demands a high level of autonomy, but good judgment is also needed – you'll have to decide when to act on your own authority and when to seek guidance. Remember, to many outside of the civil service you will be the face of officialdom.

Getting there

As I've said, to be a nursing officer, you need to have expertise and experience. In our profession, the postregistration frameworks for career development are well defined, and we have a plethora of experiential and academic provision available to us. The hard part is trying to combine full-time employment with part-time study, while balancing these with family commitments to keep a respectable work/life balance.

An alternative is to take time out of nursing to undertake full-time study. In my own case, all of my studies (excluding critical care courses and midwifery training) were undertaken as a part-time, self-funded student, until the final year of my masters degree when I was supported by my then employer who paid half of my university fees. No one can underestimate the huge commitment continuous professional development (CPD) requires if you want to succeed, and you should be realistic about this so you don't set yourself impossible goals.

no one can **underestimate** the **huge commitment** **CPD requires**

Nursing officer positions are normally advertised in the nursing press, but if you are interested in undertaking such a role it would be beneficial for you to try and get a short period of 'shadowing experience' and then you will see first hand if this is a job you would wish to pursue.

My personal approach to career planning

I would love to be able to say that I mapped out my career pathway right from the start. The truth is that as I felt I had achieved what I considered to be my optimum level of performance in a particular post, I got the urge to move on. If I stayed, I would be in danger of becoming complacent and for me personally that was wrong.

When I reached this point, I would spend time reading adverts and researching job descriptions to see what I could do next and I knew that for me to make the break from one position to the other, certain criteria had to be met: I needed to maintain clinical practice, I needed to feel challenged, I needed to aim to improve on my performance, and I needed to maintain enthusiasm and enjoy my work. It's this approach that has driven me onwards and, I guess, upwards.

The more senior I have become, the more difficult it has been to maintain clinical contact. But it's important to me that I continue to practise in a clinical environment, so I've done this in my own time, as a bank nurse, agency nurse or through an honorary contract in an acute hospital trust. This enables me to keep focused on the needs of patients and it also serves to keep me grounded as to the educational and development needs of pre-registration and postregistration nurses. Continuing clinical work also means you can engage in postregistration education and take up training opportunities.

Voice of experience
The nursing officer

- If you plan a career in government, try to secure a secondment or 'shadow' a nursing officer for a short period of time
- Work hard at your continuous professional development
- Develop networks
- Have a positive regard for colleagues and a passion to develop the profession
- Remember that when in a public role, you always have to lead by example and be beyond reproach

journalist

Tricia Reid, Former Editor of *Nursing Times*

When I was asked to write this chapter, I must admit I relished the opportunity to do a bit of public relations for the nursing press. Having edited *Nursing Times* for 4 years, a magazine that is very much at the heart of the nursing world and culture, I was often frustrated by how some nurses viewed us with fear and 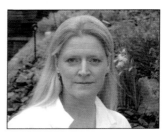 suspicion, rather than as the friend we always set out to be. This is despite the fact that *Nursing Times* has influenced policy and practice in nurses' favour for decades.

Why is that? Part of the reason is that journalists are stereotyped – even if they work for a professional title like *Nursing Times*. Like our peers on the nationals, we are often lumbered with a reputation for being duplicitous, manipulative, vainglorious twisters of the truth. We are often portrayed as having no dignity and no respect for the dignity of others, willing to destroy an individual for the satisfaction of getting the story. This stereotype was born out of the tabloid circulation wars, which began in earnest in the 1980s and which are still very much alive today.

> duplicitous, manipulative, vainglorious twisters of the truth

For most of the British press, and the professional press in particular, however, this is not the reality.

The nursing press does not exist as a propaganda machine to pass nurses off as angels. Neither does it exist to stitch them up. When I edited it, the role of *Nursing Times* was to be a voice for nurses, to stick up for them when they are getting a bad deal. But like any decent title, our job was to report the good and the bad in a way that was meaningful to our readers – nurses. Take the enquiry into the Beverly Allit murders in the mid-1990s. While the tabloids were demonizing nursing and nurses, and screaming for blood, the nursing press embarked on a soul-searching analysis, which saw nurses candidly revealing how it could easily happen again elsewhere. Readers were obviously shocked and ashamed that their profession had been called into disrepute. But the reaction was honest and human. The nursing press could not defend the indefensible. It did, however, have a role in ensuring nurses were involved in mapping a way out of the darkness.

Knowledge is power – so use it!

The media can be a powerful and wonderful thing. Good journalism can influence change in inextricable ways – depending on your point of view of course. Think of all those sleazy politicians and corrupt world leaders who have been felled by the sword of journalism. Think of how people the world over were moved to action by the powerful pictures and stories of starving Ethiopians in the 1980s. Nurses, too, can use the power of the media for the good of their profession and their own professional development. Like the world of journalism, the world of nursing has moved on. There is more pressure on nurses than ever to disseminate good practice, to prove that they are doing a good job and to demonstrate that they are active stakeholders in what promises to be the greatest reform of the health service since it was conceived in the 1950s.

Nurses are good at a lot of things. They are scientists, humanists, counsellors, advocates, guardians and communicators. Nurses are not so good at blowing their own trumpets. I could not begin to count the number of times a nurse has told me of some fascinating work she is doing and, when I asked if she had ever considered writing it up, she has shuffled her feet in that "who, little old me?" kind of way. Imagine a doctor with this attitude. Unthinkable!

nurses are not so good at blowing their own trumpets

As nurses, you are part of the biggest single group of health professionals working in the NHS. You are learning new things every day and taking on new responsibilities. You are under pressure to constantly prove yourself, to meet numerous targets and to make sure the voice of nursing is heard in every new dimension of the NHS, from primary care trusts to devising protocols for meeting the targets set out in National Service Frameworks. If you are committed to the development of an excellent health service, you know that you must communicate your ideas and learn from those of others. In an organization the size of the NHS, it is easy to become lost and alone.

I want to show you how to use the nursing media to communicate your ideas and achievements to others by getting them published. Of course, there is a price. It will mean more work, but it will be a great learning experience. You will think about your work in a different way, and you will consolidate your learning and professional development, which you should be doing anyway. And when your work is published or reported, you will have a fantastic record of it for your postregistration and practice (PREP) portfolio.

It is not necessary to shoulder the responsibility for disseminating good practice on your own. Nurses are great team players. Get your colleagues involved in documenting the team's work. Get your managers and the publicity department involved. Stop thinking of writing as a self-conscious pursuit in which some people show off and others get shown up. There is very little altruism in magazine and newspaper publishing. In general, they exist to make money and, to do that, they must publish excellent material that will make people buy them. Believe me, they will not let you look foolish.

Getting published – disseminating good practice

The need for nurses to, in the words of a former Secretary of State for Health, Alan Milburn, "pass the acid test" has already been mentioned. Basically, in this brave new world of targets, league tables, increased responsibility and multidisciplinary team working, you have got to prove that you are up to speed with the changes happening within the NHS and that you are looking to improve your practice all the time.

The environment in which you are working is a catalyst to new ways of working. Greater responsibility in areas that were previously the domain of doctors has created a whole new raft of procedures in which nurses can now get involved. Making and receiving referrals, admitting and discharging patients, and nurse prescribing are just a few examples. If you are doing something new, or something old in a new way, with demonstrable benefits for patients and staff alike, then you have a good story to tell.

Of course, there are other reasons to publish other than to tell the world you have found a good way of doing things. Academics, for example, need to publish as a matter of course and need to choose accredited journals with a research assessment exercise (RAE) rating. These journals will probably have a very small and specialist readership. Some nurses have drawn the conclusion that if the journal they publish in does not have RAE status, then it is in some way intellectually inferior. There are mixed opinions on this. My own is that if you have something worth saying that will help nurses do a better job, then you have a responsibility to disseminate it to the widest possible audience.

> go for the **widest possible audience**

How do I get started?

First, think carefully about the kind of information you want to communicate and whom you need to share it with. If it is very specialist and you feel it would only bear meaning for nurses working in the same field as you, then you may wish to consider one of the many specialist nursing journals around. The Royal College of Nursing has a number of specialist forums, many of which publish a journal for members of that forum. *The Journal of Wound Care*, published by Emap, appeals to the huge number of nurses working in that area, but is also read by practitioners working in other health disciplines. There are various specialist cancer journals and many of the nursing titles regularly publish specialist supplements.

I would advise choosing the journal that you would like to see your work published in before you begin to write. It is much easier to write for a defined audience than to try and pick a journal that suits your style. If you have had to write up the results of your work either for a course that you are on or because the trust or your manager requires it, you will have already made a good start. However, it will still require some work to turn it into an article. If you are a first timer (or even if you are not), the following guidelines will help you submit something close to what the editors can work with.

Talk to someone!

You can save a lot of wasted effort and disappointment by just lifting the phone and talking to someone at the publication you wish to submit to. Look at what the trade endearingly calls the 'flannel panel' – the names and job titles of the people who produce the magazine or journal. If your work is practice based, look for a clinical editor. If it is opinion, comment, personal experience or policy, you may find the features editor is the right person. Or you can always talk directly to the editor. Ask for the 'Guide for Contributors', which will tell you how to format the work, how long it should be and so on.

Be ready to explain your idea and answer some questions.

- Is this a new idea?
- Have you done any research into its effectiveness?
- What are the patient outcomes?
- Is it a nurse-led initiative?
- Is it something that nurses in other disciplines can learn from, or would find interesting?
- Does it respond to the demands and targets laid out in the NHS Plan?
- Could a nurse find this information elsewhere – in a textbook, for example?
- Why is it important to publish this now?

The world of nursing is certainly becoming more specialist, but do not make the mistake that, for example, a mental health nurse will not be interested in an article about nutrition. The very fact that nurses are all becoming more specialist makes it even more important to ensure good multidisciplinary working, and that you tap into the knowledge of those who know most about an area of care.

The last question is an important one. Remember publishers and editors are trying to sell their magazine – and get people to read it. If there is no immediacy, no real reason why a nurse should buy this magazine right now, then he or she will not. So we will have failed and you will have wasted your time.

When you have spoken to someone at the magazine, one of three things will happen. You will be commissioned to do some work, and given a word length, a detailed brief and a deadline. Or, if you have something already written in report form, you may be asked to send it in so that its appropriateness can be assessed. You will then get a response asking you to do further work on it. It will probably be sent out for double-blind review at this stage (you and the reviewer remain anonymous to each other). Or they will simply say no. Reasons for saying no vary. It may be that it's along the same lines as something covered recently in the title or that something similar has already been accepted. Alternatively, it may not be appropriate for the title. For example, if you want *Nursing Times* to publish your 35 000 word thesis on ingrown toenails, it will probably decline. Be realistic. If you have been looking at the magazine closely and are trying to respond to what it does, you are more likely to succeed.

Magazines also receive a number of unsolicited manuscripts. In the nursing press, however, this has dropped dramatically over the years, probably because nurses are just too busy to write something in the vague hope that someone will publish it. However, editors will appraise everything. If you do send in a piece of coursework on the recommendation of a tutor, again, be realistic. If accepted, you will certainly have to rework it.

Where is the patient?

I have read so many articles and papers in which the patient is not mentioned once. You must demonstrate that you are working *with* the patient not *on* the patient. There is nothing that breathes life into an article like a case study. Editors love them, readers love them and they are an excellent way of demonstrating what you mean. Case studies do not need to have a happy ending. If it demonstrates a learning point, all well and good. All nurses identify with case studies, even when things did not go entirely to plan. Remember that

> nothing **breathes life** into an **article** like a **case study**

the whole essence of the NHS Plan is to put the patient at the centre – and quite right too.

Always change the name of the patient described in your case study. Editors will usually check, but many will assume that you have already done so, so do not take chances.

Structure – beginning, middle and end

The beginning is very important. You must draw the reader in. "Patient re-admissions following surgery have been halved thanks to a new nurse-led discharge protocol" will grab the reader more than "Nurses at Oaktree Hospital were asked to look into developing better discharge procedures following a rapid rise in re-admissions". The first emphasizes the positive and the reader immediately knows they are going to learn how to do something better and get good results.

The middle should spell out how you did it. Tell the reader very early on the results you achieved and make comparisons with the old regimen. Describe the research that you did, what statistics you gathered, who you involved and what support you received from managers. This is also a good place to put your case studies. Spell out the obstacles and how you overcame them. Use boxes and

use boxes and tables to show statistics

tables to show statistics; they look attractive and make information easier to understand. Do not worry about presenting them in perfect form. The magazine's art team can turn very basic information into professional-looking artwork.

For your ending, draw some conclusions. If appropriate, you could summarize by providing a checklist of things to do to get a similar project off the ground. Reassert the results you gained.

You may also like to add some further reading, but try to keep references to those that really matter and ensure that they are as up to date as possible. Some people still seem to think that the more references you cite, the better the article. This is rarely so. It is not necessary to cite the code of conduct in everything.

When you are ready to submit

Send two copies, typed double-spaced and a disk. Include any illustrations or photographs if you have them. Any drawings will probably not be used in their original form, but will act as a good guideline for people commissioning quality illustrations to go with your work. Keep a copy of everything for yourself.

You may now have to play the waiting game. For a weekly title such as *Nursing Times*, publishing up to 20 clinical pages a week, the turnaround time can be quick. Less frequent titles could take longer. You should get an acknowledgement. If you have not heard anything after 4 weeks, call them.

Your work will be subject to internal and external review. When all comments have been gathered, the editor of your work will contact you.

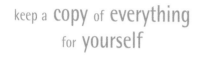

keep a **copy** of **everything** for **yourself**

Your work may be rejected at this point, but it is most likely that you will be asked for further information. If the suggested changes and additions are minor, they will probably call and discuss it with you. Major changes will be requested in writing and the revised article may well have to go through the whole review process again.

Once your article has been accepted, you should be kept involved in the production process. Your article may be cut and it will be edited. How much control you have over this depends on the publication. Most will send you first proofs, inviting comments on factual inaccuracy only. Proofs are not an opportunity to rewrite.

Selling a story

If that all sounds a bit too much like hard work, there are easier ways of getting your message across or highlighting your good practice. You could 'sell' your story to the magazine. Selling a story is a bit of a misnomer as you are unlikely to get paid unless you are doing a kiss-and-tell job on a public figure, in which case you are likely to pay with your job. So, be realistic. Tales of achievement are manna from heaven for journalists on the nursing press. If it is topical, it is even better. The government announces plans for reducing teenage pregnancies. You are working at a GP surgery where you have reduced them significantly over 2 years. Ring the news desk or the features editor. They will want to interview you!

You may have a more negative story to tell, which would be best covered impartially by a journalist. Whistle-blowing, for example, is a big issue in the NHS. Nurses have a duty to expose bad practice, particularly when it affects patient safety. This begins to stray into very sensitive territory and nurses are faced with a serious dilemma. Sticking your neck out when everyone else is burying their head in the sand is a very hard thing to do and the consequences are rarely good. But you could write anonymously to a magazine, or you could call and have an off-the-record discussion about your concerns. A good journalist will not betray you and can advise the best course of action to avoid incriminating yourself.

a good journalist will not betray you

It is a brave nurse who will come clean on bullying, violence in the workplace, work-related stress, racism or poor patient care. You need to think twice before going it alone. Get the advice and support of your union. Offering your experiences as part of a bigger campaign is always a good bet and all the nursing unions are constantly waging war on these issues. But the success of these campaigns relies on support from the media. *Nursing Times* ran a campaign called 'Stamp Out Violence' in 1998, which was to influence government policy on dealing with violence in the workplace. The nurses who told their stories should get all the credit.

A lot of lip service has been paid to whistle-blowing and sadly the reality is that support mechanisms for whistle-blowers are still wildly inadequate. Thankfully, people still feel the need to do it. And when it comes to exposing wrongdoing, the media comes into its own.

Crossing the great divide

In almost a decade of working alongside nurses, I have watched many brilliant practising nurses forsake life at the patient's bedside for a career in journalism. The nursing press is always crying out for great nurse contributors, and all of them have nurses on the staff. Their experiences as practitioners and their knowledge of what makes nurses tick is an invaluable resource.

If you are looking for a career in journalism, the chances are that you will want to utilize your experience as a nurse. You may want to do this specifically in the nursing press, or you may wish to develop a specialty in the broader issues of healthcare. If you want to cash in on your nursing experience, moving from clinical nursing into a nursing journal is not necessarily a route out of the profession – if that is what you are looking for. You will be expected to maintain your credibility as a practitioner. You may never go back to nursing, but you will be expected to think and act as if you will! You will be relied upon to keep up to date with policy developments, as well as research and clinical innovations. And on top of all that, you will be expected to be a good journalist too, able to spot a story and brimming with ideas.

> you will be relied upon to keep up to date

A lot of the skills of journalism can be taught, but in my view good journalists have a natural ability. If you have not got the bottle to pick up the phone and ask a question over and over until you get an answer, you will not enjoy journalism. You can do journalism degrees and diplomas, but any good training must be complemented by good practical experience in a real magazine or newspaper environment. Most of all, you will need a good questioning mind.

It is not easy, but neither is nursing. If the idea of a career in journalism tempts you, start working on a relationship with a magazine you like. Get writing – letters, columns, book reviews – try the lot. Ask your chosen magazine if you could do some work experience. If you are self-motivated and have a broad clinical knowledge, you will get a try. You will need passion, a go-getting attitude and a good sense of humour.

The future

Nursing is not a black and white issue. Nursing is standing on the brink of great change and it is an exciting time to be a nurse. In the NHS of the new millennium, you have to decide whether you are a player or a spectator. If you are reading this book, you have probably already decided that playing is much more fun. The opportunities to go forward are immeasurable, but to do so, nurses need their seat at the table of influence. Do not rely on a handful of nursing leaders to claim it for you. Nurses will always be judged by what they do. So use the media and tell the world!

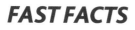
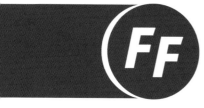

'***** outstanding'

on *Fast Facts – HIV in Obstetrics and Gynaecology*, in *Journal of Pelvic Surgery*, 2001

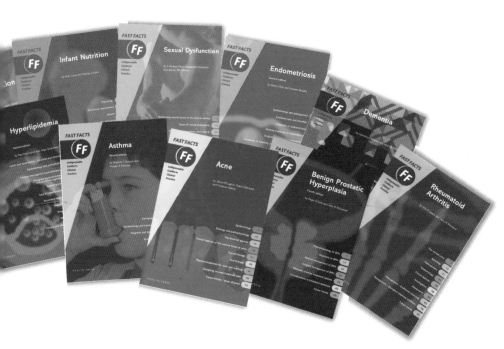

'explains the important facts and demonstrates the levels of "good practice" that can be achieved'

on *Fast Facts – Minor Surgery*, in *Journal of the Royal Society for the Promotion of Health* 122(3), 2002

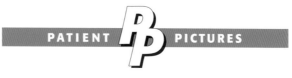
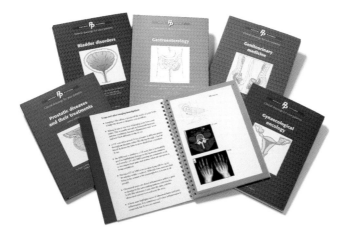

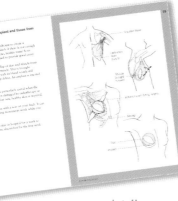

'strikes a perfect balance between comprehensiveness and accessibility'

on *Patient Pictures – Breast Cancer* in *Update*, April 2003

'It is often helpful to have pictures to help explain to the patients all about their particular problem. This book fulfils that need. ...This book will be a useful tool in a general practice surgery, family planning, antenatal, well woman, gynaecology and urology outpatients clinic'

on *Patient Pictures – Bladder Disorders* in *The Journal of the Royal Society for the Promotion of Health*, September 2000

Fast Facts

Acne

Allergic Rhinitis

Ankylosing Spondylitis

Anxiety, Panic and Phobias (second edition)

Asthma (second edition)

Benign Gynecological Disease (second edition)

Benign Prostatic Hyperplasia (fifth edition)

Bipolar Disorder

Bladder Cancer

Bleeding Disorders

Brain Tumors

Breast Cancer (third edition)

Chronic Obstructive Pulmonary Disease

Coeliac Disease

Colorectal Cancer (second edition)

Contraception (second edition)

Dementia

Depression (second edition)

Diseases of the Testis

Disorders of the Hair and Scalp

Dyspepsia (second edition)

Eczema and Contact Dermatitis

Endometriosis (second edition)

Epilepsy (second edition)

Erectile Dysfunction (fourth edition)

Gynaecological Oncology

Headaches (second edition)

HIV in Obstetrics and Gynecology

Hyperlipidemia (third edition)

Hypertension (second edition)

Infant Nutrition

Inflammatory Bowel Disease (second edition)

Irritable Bowel Syndrome (second edition)

Low Back Pain

Menopause (second edition)

Minor Surgery

Multiple Sclerosis (second edition)

Obstructive Sleep Apnea

Ophthalmology

Osteoporosis (fourth edition)

Parkinson's Disease

Prostate Cancer (fourth edition)

Prostate Specific Antigen (second edition)

Psoriasis (second edition)

Renal Disorders

Respiratory Tract Infection (second edition)

Rheumatoid Arthritis

Schizophrenia (second edition)

Sexual Dysfunction

Sexually Transmitted Infections

Skin Cancer

Smoking Cessation

Soft Tissue Rheumatology

Specific Learning Difficulties

Stress and Strain (second edition)

Superficial Fungal Infections

Travel Medicine

Urinary Continence (second edition)

Urinary Stones

Fast Facts – Highlights

Psychiatry Highlights 2003–04

Rheumatology Highlights 2003–04

Urology Highlights 2004–05

Vascular Surgery Highlights 2004–05

Patient Pictures

Breast Cancer

Cardiology

End-Stage Renal Failure

ENT

Erectile Dysfunction

Fertility

Gastroenterology

Gynaecology (second edition)

HIV Medicine

Ophthalmology

Prostatic Diseases and their Treatments
    (second edition)

Rheumatology (second edition)

Urological Surgery (second edition)

Succeeding as

Succeeding as a GP

Succeeding as a Nurse

To order: Fill in the form, complete your credit card details or enclose a cheque payable to NBN International Limited and send to: NBN International Limited, Plymbridge House, Estover Road, Plymouth PL6 7PY. Alternatively, call 01752 202301 and have your credit card details ready, fax this form to 01752 202333 or email orders@nbninternational.com. For enquiries, please fax 01752 202331.

All books are priced £15.00 For every three books you order you can choose another one for **FREE**. Please write FREE in the sub-total column of the relevant book. There are no restrictions on how many free books you can qualify for.

I would like to order:

Qty	Title	Sub-total
____	_____	_____
____	_____	_____
____	_____	_____
____	_____	_____
____	_____	_____
____	_____	_____

Postage and packing: UK: £3 for the first book and £1 each additional book / maximum charge £10.00
Export orders based on weight and destination.

TOTAL _____

Payment details

a) I wish to pay by credit card ☐ MasterCard ☐ Visa ☐ Delta ☐ Switch

I authorize you to debit my account with the amount of £ _____

Credit card number ☐☐☐☐ ☐☐☐☐ ☐☐☐☐ ☐☐☐☐

Issue number (Switch only) ☐☐☐   Expiry date ☐☐☐☐

b) I enclose a cheque for £ _____ made payable to NBN International Limited

Signature (order invalid without signature) _____

Delivery details

Title and name _____

Address _____

_____

_____

Telephone _____ Email _____

NBN International Limited • Plymbridge House • Estover Road • Plymouth • PL6 7PY
Tel: 01752 202301 • Fax: 01752 202333 (orders) / 202331 (enquiries) •
Email: orders@nbninternational.com

SAN443

succeeding
as a

nurse

Your opinion counts!

Succeeding as a nurse is for all nurses – those about to embark on a career in this caring profession and those who are already established on the path to success.

Expert authors have striven to combine a wealth of general information and practical advice with more detailed insights into the specific skills required to follow and enjoy a successful career path in modern nursing.

We hope that reading this book has made a real difference to you: to the way you view yourself and your colleagues, to your role in your chosen profession and to your future.

We would like you to help us to continue to make a difference by helping us to shape future editions of *Succeeding as a nurse*.

We invite your feedback, good and bad. Help us to help you and those who follow you into a nursing career by sending your comments to the Health Press team at: post@healthpress.co.uk

Thank you!